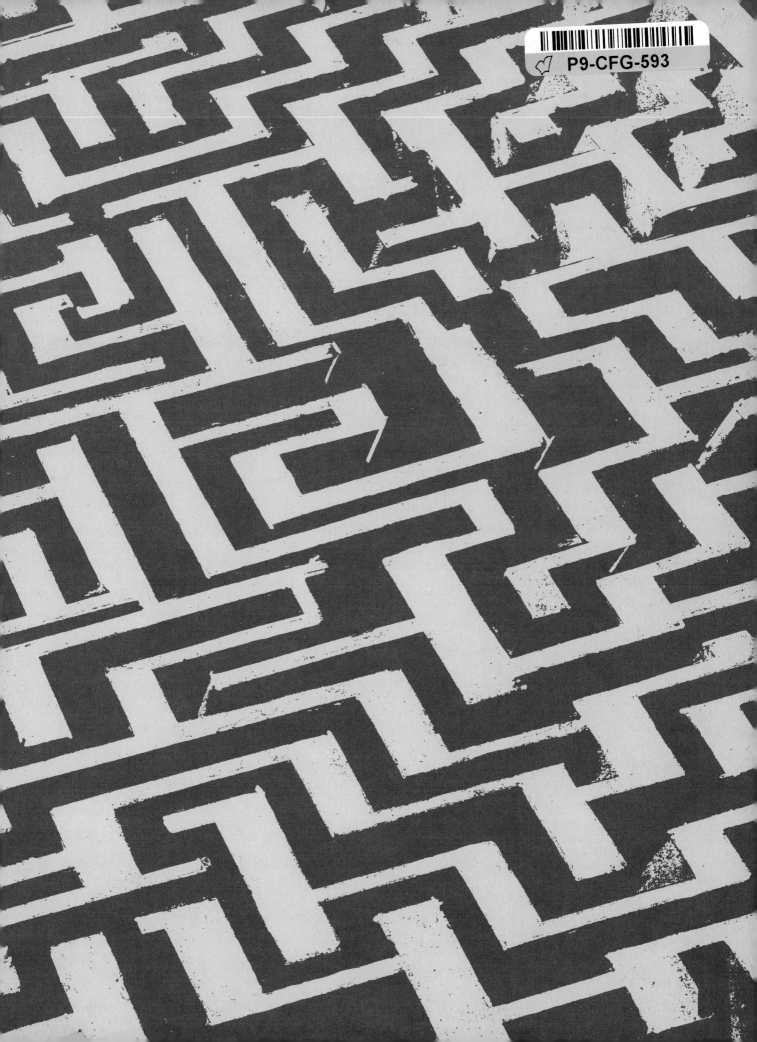

P9-CFG-593

QUEST FOR THE UNKNOWN

LIFE BEYOND
DEATH

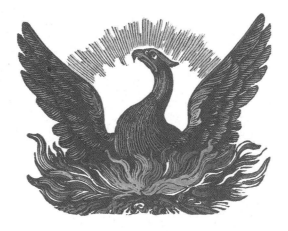

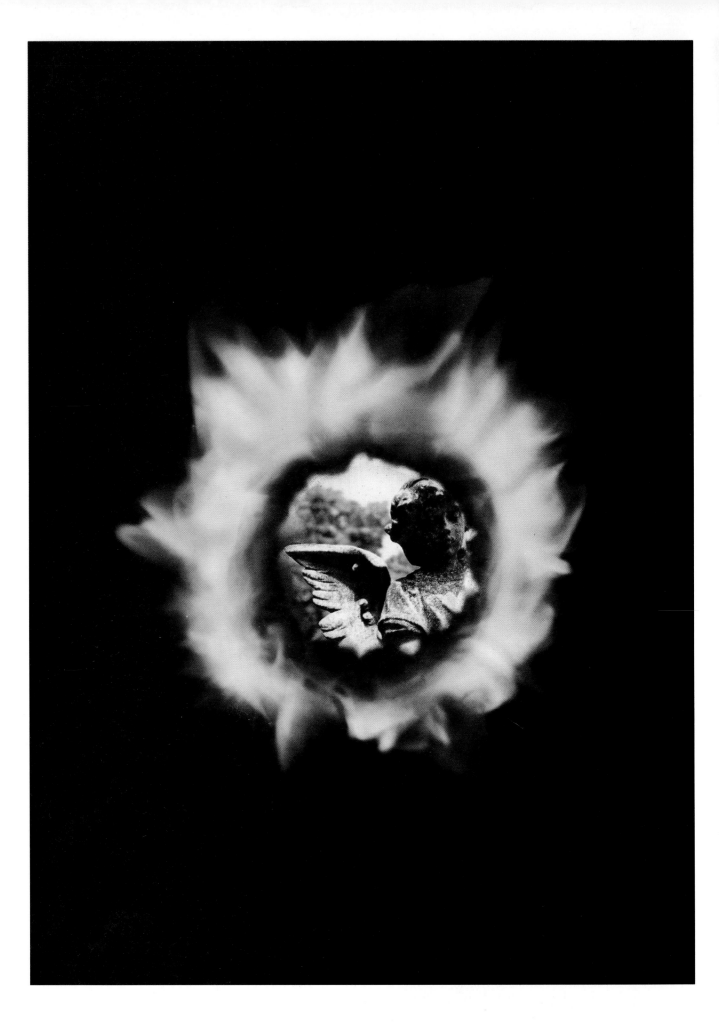

QUEST FOR THE UNKNOWN

LIFE BEYOND DEATH

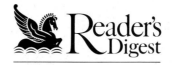

Reader's
Digest

THE READER'S DIGEST ASSOCIATION, INC.
Pleasantville, New York/Montreal

Quest for the Unknown
Created, edited, and designed by DK Direct Limited

A Dorling Kindersley Book

DK Direct Limited

Senior Editor Sue Leonard
Editors Ellen Dupont, Nance Fyson
Editorial Research Julie Whitaker
Editorial Secretary Pat White

Senior Art Editor Simon Webb
Designer Susie Breen
Picture Research Frances Vargo; **Picture Assistant** Sharon Southren

Editorial Director Jonathan Reed; **Design Director** Ed Day

Volume Consultants Reg Grant, Lynn Picknett
Contributors Vida Adamoli, David Christie-Murray, Barbara Harris,
Lynn Picknett, Roy Stemman
Illustrators Jovan Djordjevic, Roy Flooks, Printed Picture Company,
Mark Surridge, Graham Ward
Photographers Billy Carter, Simon Farnhell, Andrew Griffin,
Mark Hamilton, Steve Lyne, Susanna Price, Alex Wilson

Library of Congress Cataloging in Publication Data

Life beyond death.
      p.   cm. — (Quest for the unknown)
   Includes index.
   ISBN 0-89577-399-6
   1. Death — Miscellanea. 2. Spiritualism. 3. Future life. 4. Near
-death experiences. I. Reader's Digest Association. II. Series.
BF1275.D2L53 1992
133.9'01'3—dc20   91-25399

Printed in the United States of America

FOREWORD

*O*NE OF THE MOST PROFOUND mysteries confronting any human being is the possibility of surviving after death. Traditionally, the various organized religions have provided their followers with different versions of what they can expect from the afterlife, from the Christian concept of heaven and hell to the Buddhist belief in *nirvana*. In our increasingly secular age however, many people hold the view that this important subject should be explored altogether separately from the specific context of any religious doctrine.

Research into this matter began in earnest in the mid-19th century, spurred by reports of contact with the spirit world through mediums. Since then hundreds of apparently inexplicable cases have been painstakingly investigated in an attempt to establish conclusively whether such communication is possible. Another area of intensive scrutiny is that of psychic art: works of music, painting, or literature produced by otherwise ordinary people who claim that their hands are guided by long-dead personalities such as Beethoven, Renoir or Jane Austen.

This volume examines the impressive body of work carried out in these and many other areas of psychical research, including a relatively recent phenomenon known as the near-death experience. This term describes what sometimes happens when people who have clinically "died" are brought back to life by sophisticated medical techniques. Later, they are not only able to relate all the thoughts and feelings they experienced in the very jaws of death, but they can often describe in astoundingly accurate detail everything that went on around them when they were unconscious. It may be that cases like these, made possible by huge advances in scientific knowledge, will provide the strongest evidence yet, if not for life beyond death, then at least for the existence of a very different dimension to the world we already inhabit.

— The Editors

CONTENTS

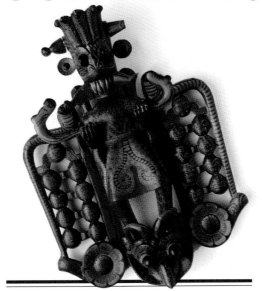

FOREWORD

5

INTRODUCTION
BEYOND AND BACK

8

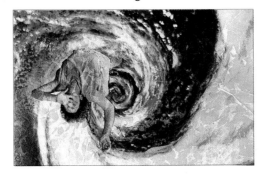

CHAPTER ONE
OUT OF THIS WORLD

18

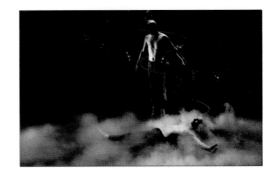

LOOKING INTO DEATH
TO HELL AND BACK
THE BRAIN'S LAST FLING
CASEBOOKS
OUT-OF-BODY EXPERIENCES
CASEBOOKS
ASTRAL TRAVEL

CHAPTER TWO
LIFE AFTER LIFE

40

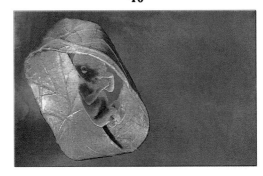

CYCLES OF REBIRTH
THE DALAI LAMA
CASEBOOKS
HYPNOTIC MEMORIES
HIDDEN EVIDENCE
FAMOUS BELIEVERS
CASEBOOKS
REINCARNATION: THE BIG DEBATE
ALTERED IMAGES
VOLUNTARY POSSESSION
CASTING OUT EVIL
A SENSE OF DÉJÀ VU
CHARTING PAST LIVES

CHAPTER THREE
DO THE DEAD SPEAK?
72

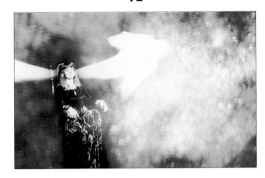

SPIRITUAL CONTACT
LINES OF COMMUNICATION
ART FROM THE PAST
CONTEMPORARY CHANNELS
FANTASTIC VISIONS
RUTH AND REALITY
GHOSTS AND TIMESLIPS
THE LAST FAREWELL

CHAPTER FOUR
DEATH: THE ENIGMA
98

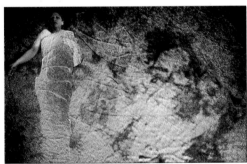
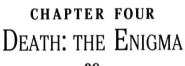

SUSPENDING LIFE
AN ACT OF WILL
FATAL ASSUMPTIONS
THE LIVING DEAD
ZOMBIES – THE WALKING DEAD

CHAPTER FIVE
AFTER THE JUDGMENT
116

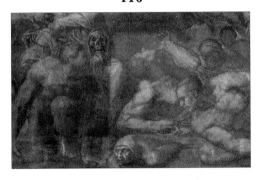

THE SPIRITUALIST ADVENTURE
POOLED RESOURCES
VISIONS OF HEAVEN AND HELL
SURVIVAL PACTS
CONCLUSIVE COMMUNICATIONS
FAMOUS LAST WORDS
AFTERLIFE REPORTING

INDEX
142

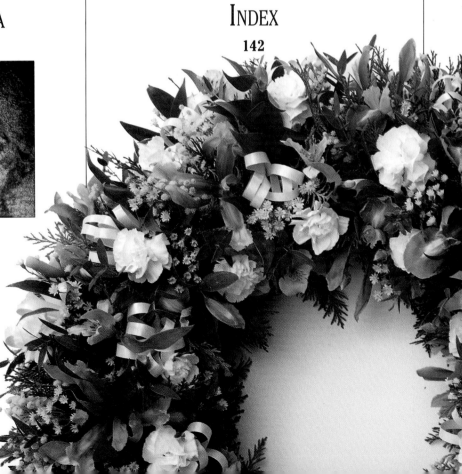

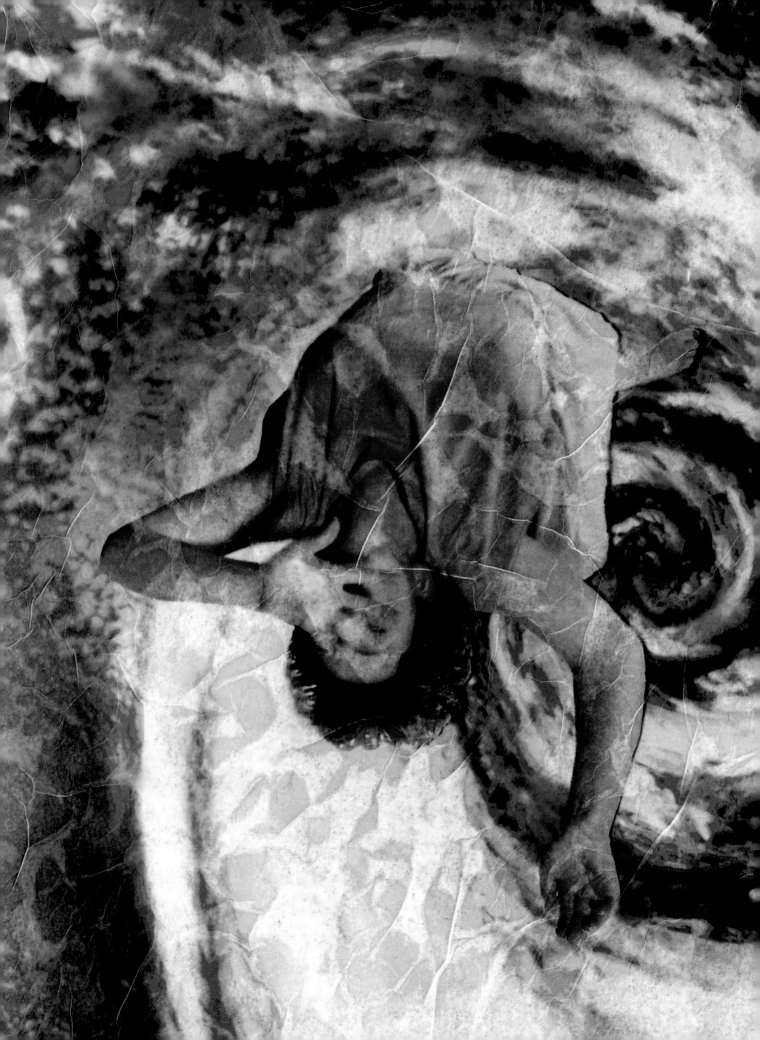

BEYOND AND BACK

The possibility of an existence after death fascinates us all. For psychics, channelers, mediums, and reincarnationists the continuation of life is a certainty. In recent years many ordinary people without mystical connections have also become convinced, having had what they believe to be an inspirational glimpse beyond the grave.

Barbara Harris, a 32-year-old housewife, had been suffering from chronic back pain for several years. Her doctors had prescribed Valium for her as a muscle relaxant, and other drugs to help ease her discomfort. Between 1973 and 1975 she was admitted to the hospital for treatment four times. A procedure called a nerve block had been performed in an attempt to deaden the sensory nerves in her lower spine, but this had proved entirely unsuccessful. During each of her admissions she had been put in traction for two weeks at a time. She became dependent on prescription drugs, and still her back pain continued. In May 1975 Barbara Harris was admitted to a Michigan hospital. Her doctors planned an exploratory and spinal fusion operation, a procedure that joins two adjacent vertebrae together in order to halt any abnormal movement that might have been causing the severe pain.

This is Barbara Harris's own account of the extraordinary events surrounding that operation.

"My life couldn't go on anymore the way it was. I wasn't able to be a mother to my children or a wife to my husband. I needed that surgery so that I could get better and return to my family. I told a chaplain who came to visit me the night before surgery, 'If there really is a God like you're telling me, then tell Him to help the surgeons fix my back or let me die. I can't go on living like this anymore!' At this time I was an atheist, a hard materialist. I didn't believe in anything beyond physical reality. And I certainly had never heard of a near-death experience.

Extensive surgery
"The surgery became much more extensive than was planned because the physicians found one vertebra totally loose. Doctors told me later it was like a child's loose tooth. Most of the loose part was removed and bone chips from my hip were grafted on. I awoke to find myself in a Stryker frame circle bed.

This is a bed made up of two large chrome hoops with a stretcher suspended in the middle. It looks very much like a Ferris wheel for one.

Recovery regime
"Three times a day the nursing staff would have to place another stretcher over me, strap me in like a human sandwich and rotate me onto my face so that my lungs could drain and the skin on my back could air. I couldn't move – the bed moved me. I was to remain suspended in this awesome bed for nearly a month. Then, when they felt I was ready, I was to be put in a full body cast from my armpits to my groin and then down my right leg to my knee.

"When I awoke after surgery I did feel some relief. The bed seemed comfortable enough, and I thought my life would start getting better.

"As the pain mounted, I started to scream, realizing that this wasn't the pain of childbirth."

"Complications set in two days later. It felt to me like my entire digestive tract had swollen up. I woke in the circle bed and saw the covers raised over my stomach. In my confusion I thought I was having another baby. As the pain mounted, I started to scream, realizing that this wasn't the pain of childbirth. It was much greater. My incisions were pulling apart, my blood pressure was dropping, and I was losing blood rapidly.

"Everyone on the staff came running to my room. They were bringing carts with equipment, bottles, pumps, and tubes. I was being hooked up and plugged in, with tubes of assorted widths and colors inserted everywhere. I was screaming with all the intense pain running through my body: 'No, let me die. Leave me alone.'"

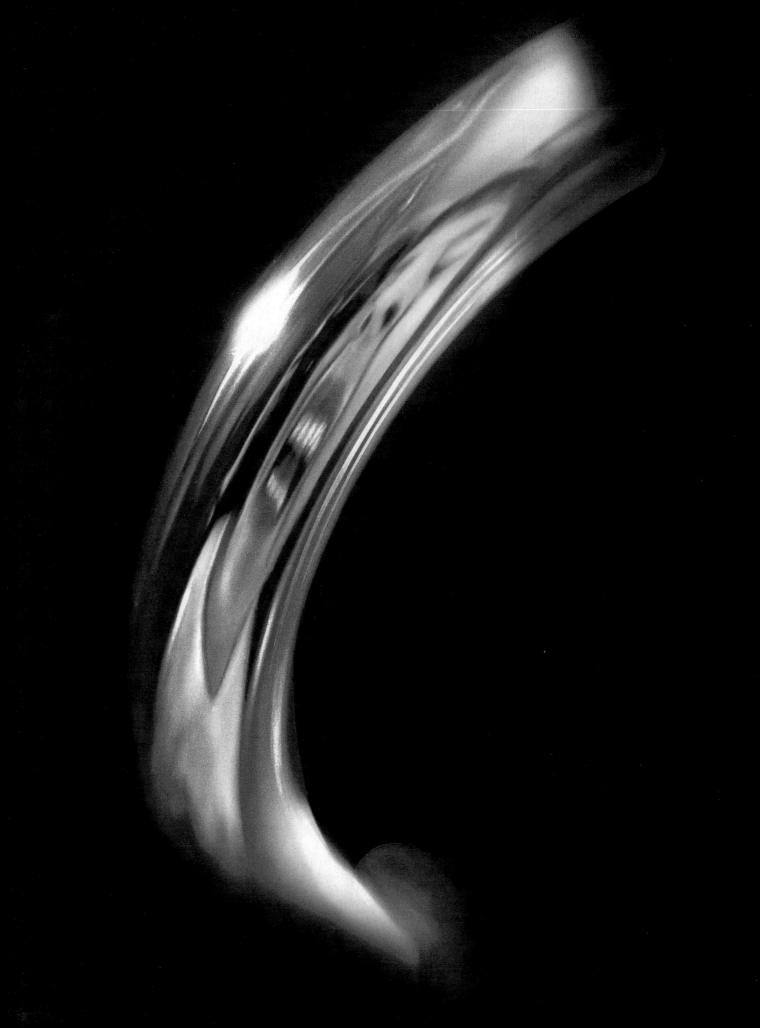

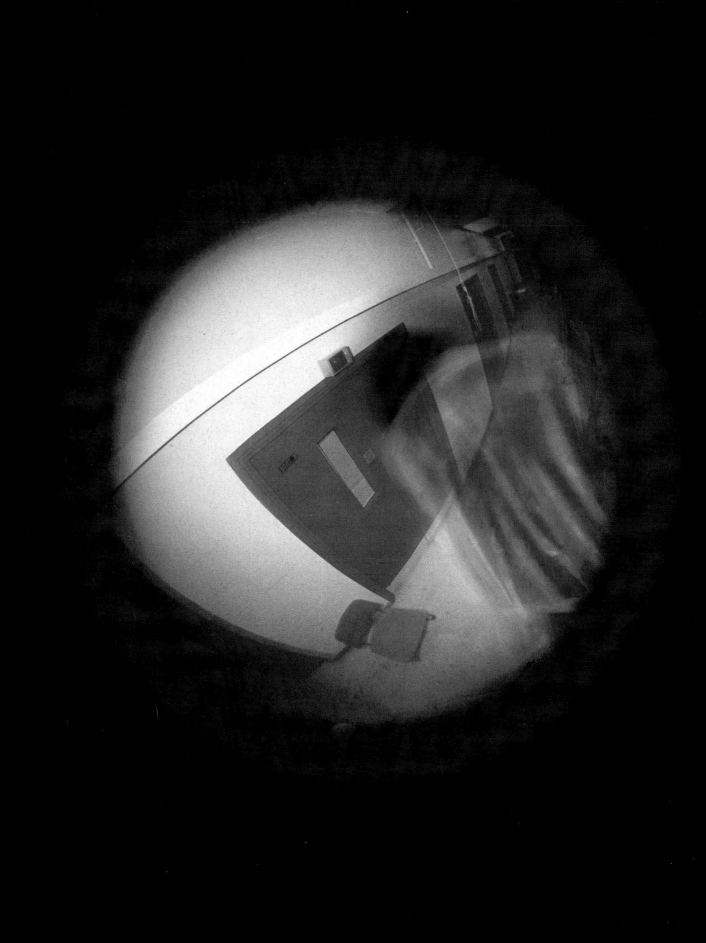

"I was in a critical, life-threatening situation. While my blood pressure plummeted and the doctors and nurses fought desperately to save me, I decided I really did want to die. I hadn't considered what would be beyond this life, but anything seemed better than drugs and casts and circle beds. As the blood drained from my body and my will to live with it, I lost consciousness.

> ## "When I had entered the hospital, the speaker was at least three feet above my head. Now, I was eye level with it."

"When I awoke, I was in the hallway of the orthopedic floor, feeling very calm and free of pain. I looked up and down the hall and saw no one. It must have been the middle of the night. I turned to go back to my room because I knew I was totally immobilized in that awesome Stryker bed and I might get into trouble if I was caught out there.

New perspective
"When I began moving back into my room, I was startled by the P.A. speaker above the doorway. I found myself looking directly into it. When I had entered the hospital, the speaker was at least three feet above my head. Now, I was eye level with it. I knew at that moment that something strange was happening. I moved back into my room and had a clear view of my body still lying in the circle bed.

External view
"'I look funny with that tape wrapped around my nose!' I said to myself. The idea of being up near the ceiling and watching myself in bed didn't confuse me at all. The only awareness I had was of how bad I looked in the bed and how well I felt for the first time in two years. I

have no idea how long I lingered up near the ceiling, but I next found myself in total blackness. 'Either my eyes aren't working or I'm in darkness,' I thought. It never occurred to me that my eyes were in my body, which was still lying in the circle bed.

Familiar embrace
"Soon, I felt drawn to someone. I was being pulled in tight. The warmth surrounded me and I recognized that wonderful childhood feeling of my grandmother pulling me close. Her bosom was huge and I felt her softness and warmth whenever she held me. No matter what I had done as a child, when she held me, I knew everything was all right. And now she was holding me again, conveying that same feeling to me. She had been dead about 13 or 14 years, but I somehow had no problems with that. I knew I was with her and we were together. I didn't believe that people existed after death, but that had nothing to do with what I was experiencing. I knew my grandmother was there. She held me for quite a while. There were no words spoken. It was an instant way of remembering and loving each other. It was all coming back for both of us. There was a wonderful feeling of merging. She was loving me the way she had always loved me.

I started moving away from my grandmother. At the same time I became aware that the blackness was churning. I was intrigued because there was light separating from it. The light was moving down, ahead of me in the same direction I was moving. It was forming, collecting, becoming the wonderful light that emanates love. I was moving toward it, and as I did so I became fascinated by my hands. It felt like they were expanding. I could feel a gentle breeze, although I couldn't see my body. There was a low droning noise drawing me towards the light.

A real experience

"Then it was morning and I was back in my body, once again trapped in the circle bed. Two nurses came in and opened the drapes at the window. I asked them to close the drapes as my eyes were very sensitive to light. My hearing seemed more acute as well. I told the staff that I had left the bed. Everyone said I was hallucinating. Only one of the doctors was willing to stop and listen intently.

Return to the darkness

"A week later, it happened again. This time I was face down in the circle bed. Lying in that position was increasingly uncomfortable because I weighed so little. Nurses always put pillows underneath me to reduce the feeling of discomfort.

"For some reason, my day nurse didn't come back after a half-hour. I realized that the nurse's call button wasn't pinned to the sheet the way it usually was in case I wanted help. I started calling out for someone to come and rotate me. I also needed the bedpan. After calling for a long time, I started screaming and then I became very hysterical.

Sobbing deeply, I separated from my body. This time I was awake and saw and felt it happen. My body in that awesome bed was moving away from me. I was back in the huge darkness.

"In the darkness was a bubble and within it the circle bed. I was still in it, crying. I saw my nurse come in and realize what had happened. She became upset and ran for help.

"Out in the darkness, above and to my left, was another bubble. In it I was a baby, about a year old. I was in my crib crying, just as much as the 32-year-old was crying in the other bubble. I looked back and forth a few times, feeling extremely confused.

"Then I realized that there was a 'presence' with me. It was certainly not an old man with a long white beard. I had given up that image when still a child. This presence was different but somehow I knew it was the same. It felt like an energy that was supporting me. It loved me just as my grandmother did – only it felt a million times stronger. The feeling was the same as the light I had sensed. It seemed an energy or a force field. The presence was infinitely huge and I was only a tiny part of it. Then suddenly our roles reversed and it was minute and part of me.

"As I moved toward the bubbles, it wasn't just me that I was feeling. I experienced my mother and my father and the person who was my boyfriend and then went on to become my husband. I could even sense what my own children were feeling. Strange as this all sounds, I didn't end at my skin. We were all one being. And the special energy was with us.

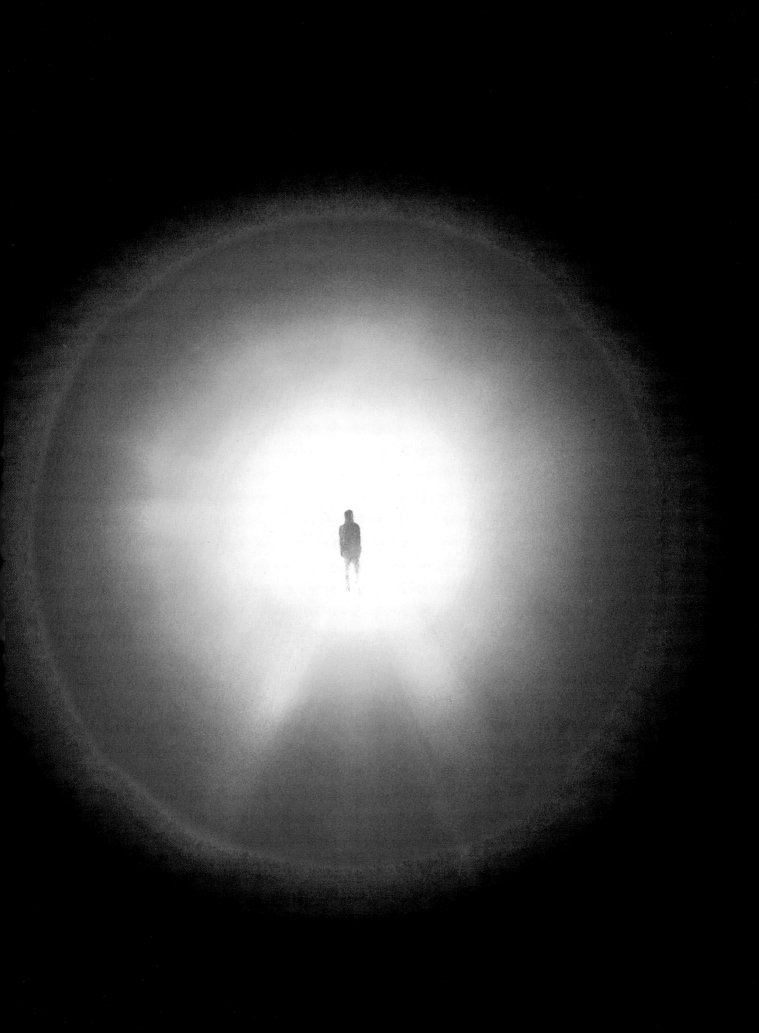

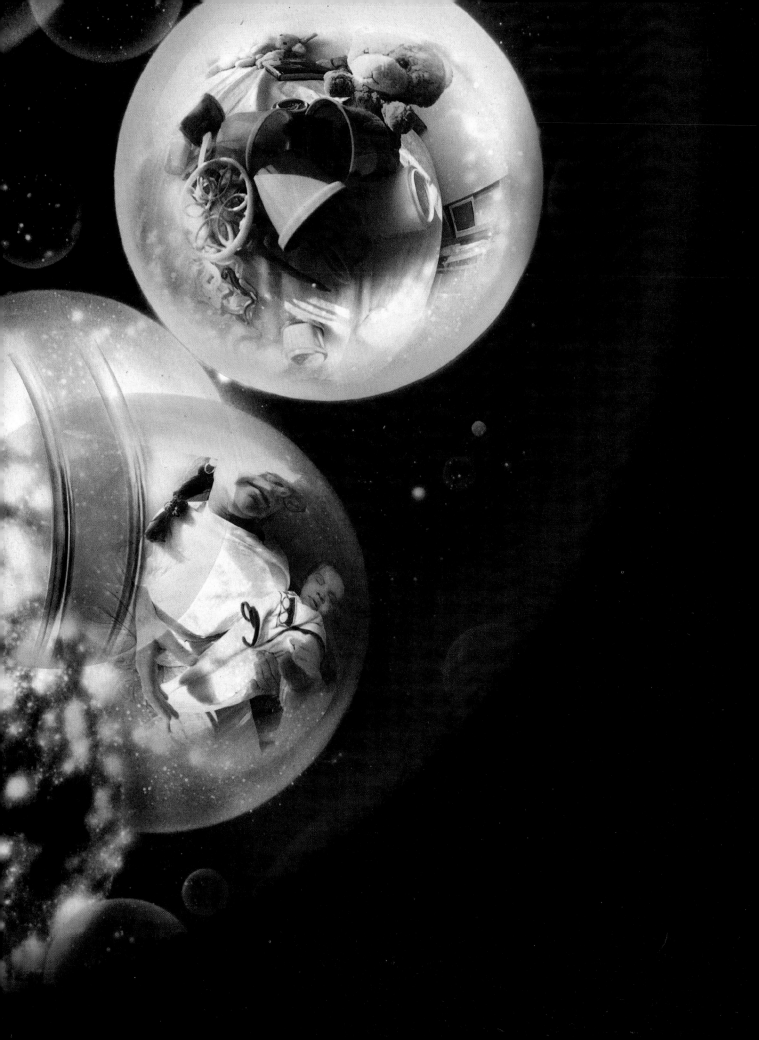

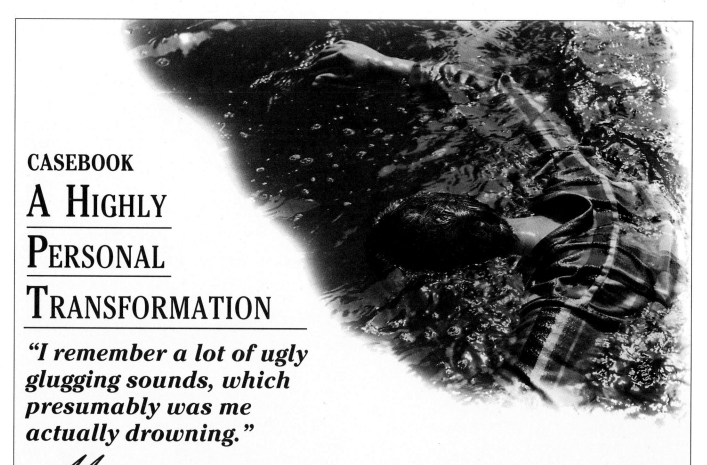

A HIGHLY PERSONAL TRANSFORMATION

"I remember a lot of ugly glugging sounds, which presumably was me actually drowning."

MANY RETURNED NEAR-DEATHERS report undergoing a completely transformed outlook on what is left of their lives. For example, atheists who thought that death was the end feel they know from experience that this is not so. Some people who held extreme religious views come to realize that heaven is not an exclusive club for their particular sect and that judgment may not necessarily be as harsh as they had been led to expect.

Day of judgment

As one man told researcher and author D. Scott Rogo: "My religion led me to believe that when you die you are met with a list of your wrongdoings and expected to make amends. I was always so frightened of death because of this. But when I had my NDE I was so overcome with love....I was turned inside out. When I came back I couldn't believe I could have been so wrong. Now I know what the phrase 'God is love' really means. I am really sorry for people who think death is pitiless and terrifying."

Going under

The idea of the NDE as being something very personal and private is repeated many times by those who have experienced it. They feel torn between the desire to share the good news and the difficulty of describing the indescribable. Carl D., from New York City, had an NDE when he was in his early twenties, and will only discuss what happened with those who are unlikely to be skeptical about it. During a fishing trip with a friend, Carl D. fell, hit his head, and drowned.

"I remember a lot of ugly glugging sounds, which presumably was me actually drowning. Then the murky old river changed into sort of bands of iridescent light, different colors, and the water was no longer wet. I found myself floating up...getting more and more ecstatic. I surfaced at an island where I sat on the sand, very happy just to sit there. Then a man came along and sat with me and I have never been so happy in my life. I suppose it was Jesus.

"Then he said I had to go back and I thought he was joking. There was a whooshing sound and I woke up being given the kiss of life and spouting filthy water. Boy, was I glad I drowned, though!"

Private beliefs

Carl D. is in no doubt that his NDE is the pinnacle of his life, a precious insight into reality. But he has learned the hard way not to try to tell everyone about it. Not only has he been mocked and ridiculed, but even those who are broadly sympathetic find it difficult to come to terms with his powerful experience. For someone who has not been there, it may be hard to fully accept the reality of such an experience.

"It's like trying to describe a beautiful painting without knowing the names of the colors. But that's only an idea of the difficulty of talking about the NDE. I guess in the end it's just something very incredible that happens between you and God."

OUT-OF-BODY
EXPERIENCES

"I felt I had left my body and...viewed it from the other side of the room. I can sort of remember looking back at myself — it was very scary."
Quoted by Dr. Kenneth Ring in *Life at Death*

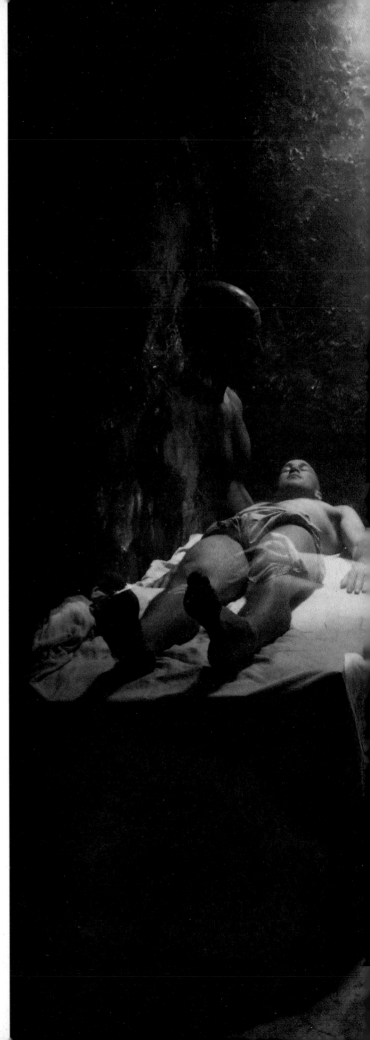

ALMOST EVERY REPORTED near-death experience includes an out-of-body experience (OBE), apparently occurring just after clinical death. Typically, people undergoing an OBE feel themselves separating from their physical body and floating above it. The detailed scenes that patients report observing during these alleged journeys out of their own bodies provide researchers with some of the strongest objective evidence for the strange reality of the whole near-death experience.

Hospital visitor

The German cancer specialist Dr. Josef Issels recorded an OBE involving an elderly woman close to death in his clinic in Bavaria, Germany.

While making his rounds one morning, Dr. Issels approached the woman's bed and greeted her in the usual way. The woman returned his greeting, then said to him: "Doctor, do you know that I can leave my body? I will give you proof, here and now." She paused for a moment, then continued: "If you go to Room 12 you will find a woman writing a letter to her husband. She has just completed the first page. I've just seen her do it." She then described in great detail what she claimed to have seen.

Issels walked to Room 12. "The scene inside was exactly the same as the woman had described it," he wrote, "even down to the contents of the letter. I went back to the elderly woman to seek an explanation. In the time I had gone she had died."

Escape from pain

Out-of-body experiences are not necessarily associated with the onset of death, however. They have been reported after a blow to the head, during a period of unconsciousness, in sleep, or at times of acute mental or physical stress. During the Second World War, British secret agent Odette Hallowes found out-of-body experiences of vital help during the desperate periods of agonizing torture she suffered at the hands of the Gestapo. Although unable to escape entirely the horrors she experienced, Hallowes found that when pain reached a peak she could rise above her physical consciousness and view the scene from a distance with a profound sense of detached relief.

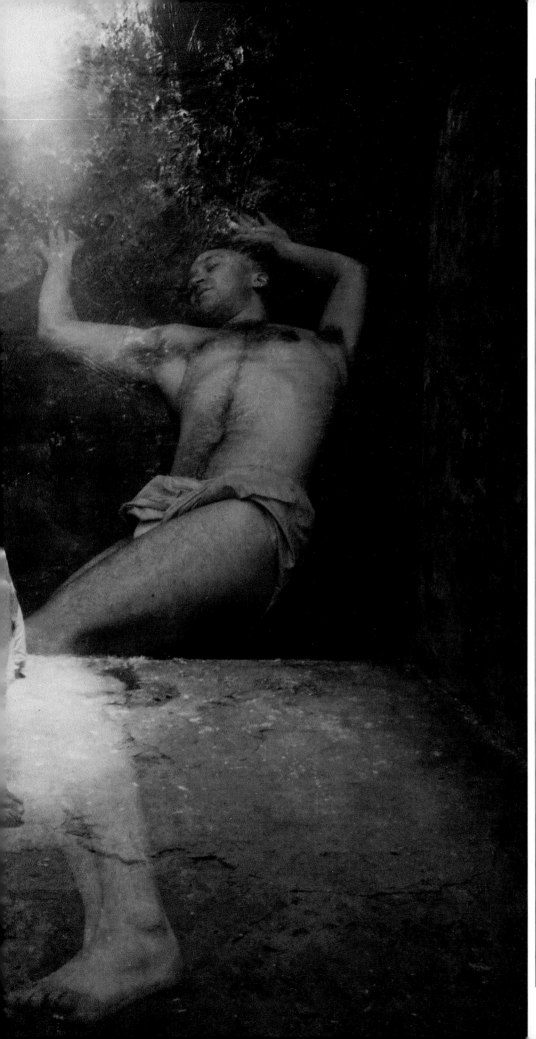

SKEPTICISM AND BELIEF

English psychologist Dr. Susan Blackmore has a particular interest in OBE's because she has experienced them herself. For example, she has described how she once found herself floating on the ceiling, looking down on her "other" self. She felt herself rise out of the room and over roofs and chimneys "before flying on to more distant places...."

Yet Dr. Blackmore believes her own experience to have been a hallucination, a view confirmed by checking the facts of her vision. In her flight she "saw" red rooftops below her, where the roofs were in fact gray. And the chimneys she had seemingly flown over proved definitely not to exist.

Medical views

A variety of possible scientific explanations have been offered for the OBE. One theory sees it as a form of lucid dreaming, in which the dreamer is asleep but at the same time conscious of dreaming. Alternatively, the OBE could be a form of hypnagogic image — the very realistic dream visions quite commonly experienced by people just on the point of falling asleep.

Blackmore herself feels the most that can be said of OBE's is that they are an altered state of consciousness with some as yet unspecified physiological basis.

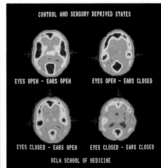

Brain scans

OBE's are especially common when people are cut off from input from the outside world through sensory deprivation. These scans show the effects of different forms of sensory withdrawal on areas of the brain.

Some people even claim the ability to fly out of the body at will, without the stimulus of any extreme stress or injury. This deliberate practice of spiritual journeying is sometimes known as astral travel. Perhaps the most famous modern practitioner of this art is Robert Monroe. In the 1970's, Monroe founded an organization in Virginia, the Monroe Institute for Applied Sciences, where the OBE technique could be taught to enthusiastic beginners.

If the claims of astral travelers are true, theirs could be a very useful talent. British psychic researcher Lynn Picknett reports the case of Yolande, who said she was capable of "popping out" for a wide variety of purposes, including escaping from the intolerable boredom

of some meetings. "I say to myself, I wonder what's on the other side of that wall, and suddenly I'm floating out of my body looking down at all the others in the meeting. Then I float off through the office or the house and have a good look round. Sometimes I've checked — in the body — that what I've seen is really there. It always is."

Experimental travel

It is possible to regard such claims with considerable skepticism, especially when anonymity protects subjects from investigation. But many experiments — often informal arrangements between friends — have purported to show that out-of–body traveling does exist, and touches on objective reality.

Picknett also recorded the case of Deidre from Leeds, West Yorkshire, England. Deidre decided to try to "travel" to the London home of a lecturer she had recently met and see if she could report back. The next day she wrote to the lecturer: "I found the area where you live on a map of London — and that's all the 'research' I did. I then went off....It

> ## "Suddenly I'm floating out of my body looking down at all the other people in the meeting."

seems to me that you live in a very small flat, down a couple of steps. There's something odd and round in the hall. It feels like rubber. It 'gives' if you put your weight on it. In your main room there is an animal. Not alive but not stuffed. Whitish. Farmyard, I think."

The lecturer admitted that she did live in a very small basement flat; that in her hall there was a minitrampoline (an indoor jogger); and that in the living room there was a large seat in the form of a sheep. Interestingly, Deidre described the sensation of putting her weight on the trampoline, yet surely an astral body has no weight. Even if the evidence in this

Astral artist
Ingo Swann claims to have made numerous psychic voyages, some into the depths of outer space. His paintings are based on his experiences during these extraordinary astral travels.

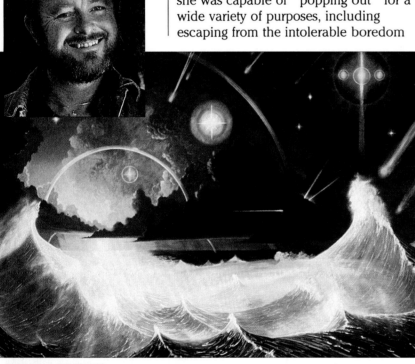

REMOTE VIEWING

It is almost impossible to construct an experiment to test the objective evidence for OBE's, because they cannot be readily distinguished from telepathy or extrasensory perception (ESP).

Consider the phenomenon known as remote viewing. In remote viewing experiments, the subject, who is usually a person of known psychic abilities, remains at "base" while an "observer" and a colleague drive to a secret location. Once there, they stroll around and talk about whatever they may see.

Back at base, the subject describes whatever comes into his or her mind. The actual location visited by the observer and the subject's recorded impressions are then checked against each other. A high

proportion of experiments conducted on these lines have produced matching information from subject and observer.

One of the most successful remote viewers is Ingo Swann, a psychic and an artist. Swann became so proficient that he could describe locations on the basis of nothing more than a set of map coordinates. The question is: Could Swann look at the map coordinates and receive an impression of the place, or did he have to travel there to look around?

case, where the participants remain anonymous, is accepted as valid, it remains impossible to confirm that an OBE was responsible. Extrasensory perception (ESP) or other psychic abilities could be involved.

There have been several interesting attempts to test claims of out-of-body travel under laboratory conditions. One of the most remarkable of these

> # Whether the out-of-body experience is actually a hallucination or a real physical occurrence remains to be established.

experiments took place at the University of California in the 1960's. A young woman, whose case reference name was Miss Z., had a reported history of OBE's since childhood. She was subjected to rigorous tests by parapsychologist Dr. Charles Tart. For four nights, Miss Z. was wired up to an electroencephalogram (EEG) at the university's sleep laboratory. The leads had been specially shortened so that she could not get up from the bed without disturbing the equipment. A slip of paper with a randomly selected number written on it was placed on a shelf above the bed. Miss Z. would only be able to read the number by leaving her own body.

On the fourth night, Miss Z. succeeded in reading out the number to the doctors in the next room. She noted that the clock above the shelf read 5:50 A.M. when she began her OBE and 6:00 A.M. when she finished it. The EEG revealed disturbed brain activity at precisely 5:57 A.M. The brain patterns on the EEG were very unusual: they could be categorized neither as sleeping nor waking.

A possible flaw

This experiment remains one of the most convincing examples of an OBE ever recorded. But, disturbingly, the parapsychologist found a possible flaw in it. Working with a colleague in the sleep chamber, he found that by flashing a light off the clockface at certain angles, it was possible to see the slip of

paper with the number written on it reflected in the clock above the bed. Tart had no reason to suspect that Miss Z. took a flashlight into the room. In fact, as far as he knows, she did not. But fraud was a possibility. There is, however, no explanation for the unusual brain waves recorded during Miss Z.'s OBE.

Skeptics such as Dr. Susan Blackmore claim that OBE's are merely products of disturbed functioning of the brain. According to this view, the sensation of floating or flying outside the physical body is all in the mind.

Certainly the information allegedly acquired by out-of-body methods can rarely be verified. Even when verification is possible, as in the case of Miss Z., the results are impossible to distinguish from ESP or telepathy.

What is true, however, beyond any reasonable doubt, is that the *experience* of floating out of the body happens to many quite normal individuals. Whether this experience is actually a hallucination or a real physical occurrence remains to be established.

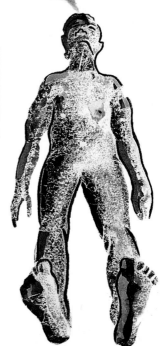

The silver cord
In occult lore the astral body is connected to the physical body by a silver cord, emerging from the third eye — the spiritual center of the body. This idea is taken from Ecclesiastes 12, where the transition from life to death is likened to the breaking of a silver cord.

FLOATING VISIT

Occasionally there are reports of OBE's in which the astral traveler is actually visible to another person.

On the night of January 26, 1957, 26-year-old Martha Johnson dreamed that she floated to her mother's house 926 miles away.

Kitchen scene
When Martha arrived there, she found her mother in the kitchen and watched what she was doing. Her mother did not seem to notice her at first, but then became aware of her standing there in a characteristic pose, with her arms folded and her head tilted to one side. Martha took a few paces toward her mother —and then woke up. She looked at the clock by her bed and saw that it was exactly 2:10 A.M.

A few days later a letter arrived from her mother, saying how she had seen Martha in her kitchen. Apparently, the moment the

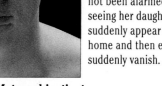

mother started to speak to her, Martha had vanished. At that point too, the family's dogs had rushed up to the kitchen door and started sniffing excitedly. In her letter she remarked favorably on her daughter's new hairstyle. She wrote that the incident had happened at "ten after two, your time."

A strong bond
Unlike other cases, which are often associated with feelings of foreboding, this one was happy. Martha's mother had not been alarmed at seeing her daughter suddenly appear in her home and then equally suddenly vanish.

Maternal instinct
In this particular story it may have been because there was a strong bond between mother and daughter that the feelings associated with the incident were entirely positive, comforting, and reassuring.

A COLORFUL LANDSCAPE

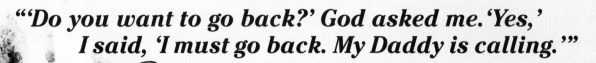

"'Do you want to go back?' God asked me. 'Yes,' I said, 'I must go back. My Daddy is calling.'"

ONE OF THE most difficult aspects of the NDE to explain away is information given to the near-deather that he or she could not have discovered in any other way. A case in point is the near-death experience of Durdana Khan, who at the age of two in 1968 "died" for 15 minutes while suffering from a mysterious neural illness. During her NDE, Durdana encountered several relatives, including one whose appearance she could not possibly have recognized.

Durdana's father was a doctor in the Pakistani Army, stationed with his family at an isolated unit in the Himalayas. Durdana's condition had been steadily deteriorating for several months, and her father was not surprised when she seemed to lose the fight for life following a particularly bad 24 hours. He tried frantically — and, in the end, successfully — to resuscitate her, calling, "Come back, my child, come back!" Durdana remembered this clearly on her return: "I heard my Daddy calling me....I told Grandpa that Daddy was calling me and I must go back. He said we should have to ask God....'Do you want to go back?' God asked me. 'Yes,' I said, 'I must go back. My Daddy is calling.'"

Vivid images

After her traumatic experience, the little girl began to talk about her time spent "with God." She described being in a beautiful garden, with white, blue, and green streams. During her first visit to some relatives, she picked out a photograph of her great-great-grandmother, saying: "This is Grandpa's grandmother. I met her in the stars." While she had never even seen a photograph of the woman, she managed to identify her immediately and correctly. Some years later Durdana was inspired to paint pictures of what she had seen when she was with God. When they were shown on British television in the early 1980's, a viewer immediately recognized the landscapes. "My God," she said, "I've been there...." She, too, believed that she had visited the garden during an NDE.

A HAPPY ACCIDENT

"I saw a light at the end of the tunnel and began to feel incredibly happy....I could see this man standing there.... I laughed, 'You're Jesus, aren't you?' I said."

WITHOUT WARNING, THE TRUCK in front stopped dead and the 26-year-old motorcyclist was thrown off his vehicle into the path of an oncoming car. He bounced off its hood and lay awkwardly on the road. People came running and someone sent for an ambulance — but there seemed to be no point. The young man was clearly dead.

"I found myself looking down on the scene from about the height of the truck. I saw the body and the white faces of the people as they realized what had happened. Actually, I only hung about until the ambulance arrived because I got bored."

Darkest fears

These are the words of Alex Thompson of Reading, Berkshire, England, whose apparently dead body was carried into the ambulance in August 1987. He describes a classic NDE: "It was as if I'd only taken half a step away from the scene of the accident when I found I was being pulled by some invisible force at an incredible speed toward a small black dot that turned into a tunnel. Although it was pitch black in there, I wasn't remotely frightened, which is odd because normally I don't like the dark much.

"I saw a light at the end of the tunnel and began to feel incredibly happy; sort of bubbly inside. By the time I got to the end, I could see this man standing there. Somehow he seemed terribly familiar to me and grinned at me. I found myself falling about laughing. 'You're Jesus, aren't you?' I said."

Alex and his heavenly companion went for a walk in a beautiful garden, but then he was told he had to return to his earth life. Although he begged to be allowed to stay, he was told he must return. He found himself being pulled back down the tunnel and came to in the emergency room, in great pain with head, back, and leg injuries. "Since that day I have absolutely no fear of death....I know I went to heaven and that it's real. It's this place that's the problem! I used to joke with friends that I was recovering from my death, but really in a sense I didn't want to.

A new beginning

"My NDE totally transformed me. Before that accident I thought God was a joke. I used to spend all my time taking my bike apart and criticizing my boss. The only future I cared about was getting drunk on holiday.

"Now I greet every day with a sense of wonder. I've started noticing things like the dew on flowers. I know it sounds corny, but it's so stunningly beautiful — yet not a patch on what heaven is like.

"And I talk to Jesus all the time, just like we did in the garden. We still joke a lot. We're the best of mates."

Like many other near-deathers, Alex has had to re-evaluate his standards. "It's like I was given a look at my life and I thought, how can I be so stupid?" he says. "I've started thinking about what I can do to help people. Maybe just getting them to understand that there's nothing to worry about is a start."

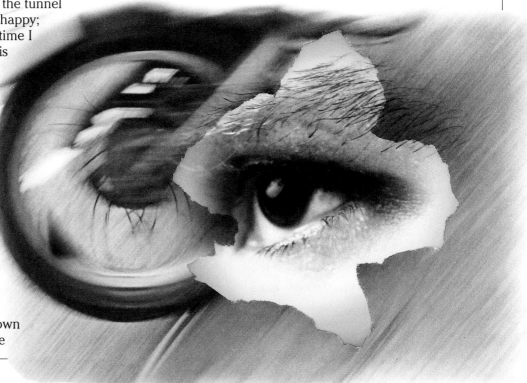

ASTRAL TRAVEL

Throughout history, out-of-body experiences (OBE's) have been sought by mystics, shamans, and holy men as a form of contact with other worlds.

A TRAVEL GUIDE

The classic work *The Projection of the Astral Body* by Sylvan Muldoon and Hereward Carrington, published in 1929, contains a wealth of practical advice for aspiring astral travelers. They believed a combination of

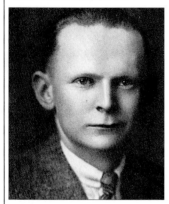

Sylvan Muldoon

imagination and willpower would achieve the desired results.

Muldoon and Carrington advised their readers to try and imagine that their astral body was rotating on the ceiling, or to try going to bed thirsty and sending the astral body downstairs for a cooling drink of water.

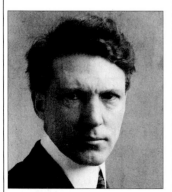

Hereward Carrington

Those who attempted to follow the authors' advice often reported strange experiences, including the sensation of flying. But most psychologists believe this simply provides interesting evidence for the power of self-hypnosis.

OBE's HAVE BEEN induced deliberately through a variety of rituals and practices. The fakirs of India and the monks of Tibet claimed to know how to produce such flights out of the body through the mortification of the flesh. The term "astral travel" has been coined for a consciously sought-after OBE.

Some believers in astral travel assert that a human being has both a physical body and another that is astral, or ethereal. This astral body is an exact copy of its physical equivalent, but made of a much more refined material. Under certain circumstances, the astral body can separate itself from the physical body and move about freely in the "astral plane." This is a space that includes the material world and also stretches beyond it. In death, the astral body detaches itself from the flesh-and-blood self forever.

Dangerous journey

As well as forming a part of the beliefs and practices of many ancient religions, astral travel has been an object of great curiosity for modern psychic researchers. There is a school of thought that warns against any such experiments, however. If the soul is out of the body, even temporarily, then the body may be taken over by another spirit, perhaps evil. In other words, the vacancy in the body may allow it to be "possessed." Or something may happen to prevent the astral body from returning to its physical double, which will then die. Whether a reality or a hallucination, the experience of astral travel has been described by some who have experienced it as terrifying.

Sacred flights

Shamans are holy medicine men traditionally revered by North American Indians and other tribesmen, from the wilds of Siberia to the Amazonian jungle. The medicine men have claimed the ability to fly out of their bodies when in a state of trance. On these flights the shamans allegedly commune with supernatural beings, or escort the spirits of the dead to the afterworld.

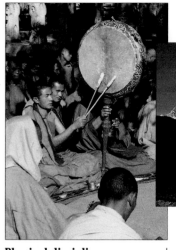

Physical discipline

In their Tibetan monasteries Buddhist monks seek spiritual powers through the strict control of the body. By subjecting themselves to intense cold or fasting, they hope to achieve a mental state in which the spirit quits the body — a form of astral travel.

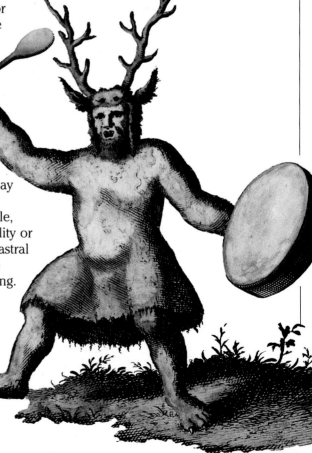

Tartar shaman

Witching ways

The power of flight was an essential attribute of a medieval witch. It was claimed that the witches flew through the air — sometimes on broomsticks — to their unholy witches' sabbaths. There they met the devil, who had the shape of a monstrous goat, and partook of human flesh. The evidence for these evil happenings comes from confessions obtained under torture, yet many hundreds of such descriptions publicized during witch trials showed a remarkable consistency. Some modern researchers believe witches may really have experienced the sensation of flying through the use of a hallucinogen, such as bufotenin. This is a natural secretion of the toad that may have been applied to the skin as a magical "flying ointment."

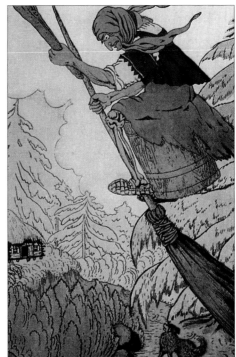

A witch astride a broomstick

BIRD OF DEATH

According to interpretations of their tomb paintings, the ancient Egyptians had a highly developed notion of the astral plane. They believed it could be entered from the physical world by any of 10 portals or 7 doors.

The Egyptians represented the astral body by a hawk with a human head, the ba. This is sometimes shown standing behind a living person, and sometimes hovering above a mummified corpse.

No one can now know whether ancient Egyptians based their belief in the astral body on their direct experience of OBE's, or whether their mythology was a complicated fiction expressing collective fears and aspirations.

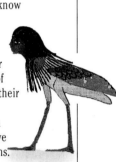

The common toad

Magic root

The mandrake is a forked root resembling the human form. The root was considered magical in medieval times. This may have been because it contains hyoscyamine — a drug that gives the illusion of flight. If it is taken in excess, hyoscyamine can cause insanity.

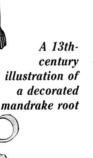

A 13th-century illustration of a decorated mandrake root

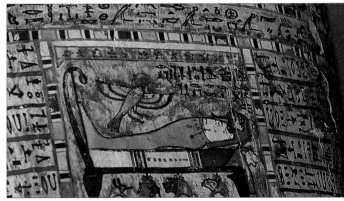

"The Soul Hovering Above the Body," by William Blake

Blake's vision

The English poet, painter, and visionary William Blake represented the soul of a dying man as a female form escaping from his body. Much of Blake's work is known to have been based on his own visionary experiences. It has been suggested that the poet underwent OBE's and that this illustration is a reliable reconstruction of them.

The flight of ba
This coffin lid, from 200 B.C., vividly depicts the ancient Egyptian image of the ethereal soul leaving the physical body.

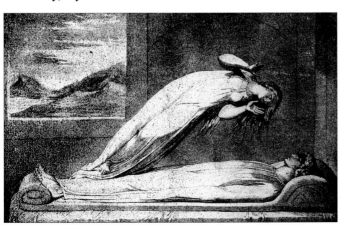

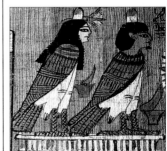

Egyptian representations of astral bodies

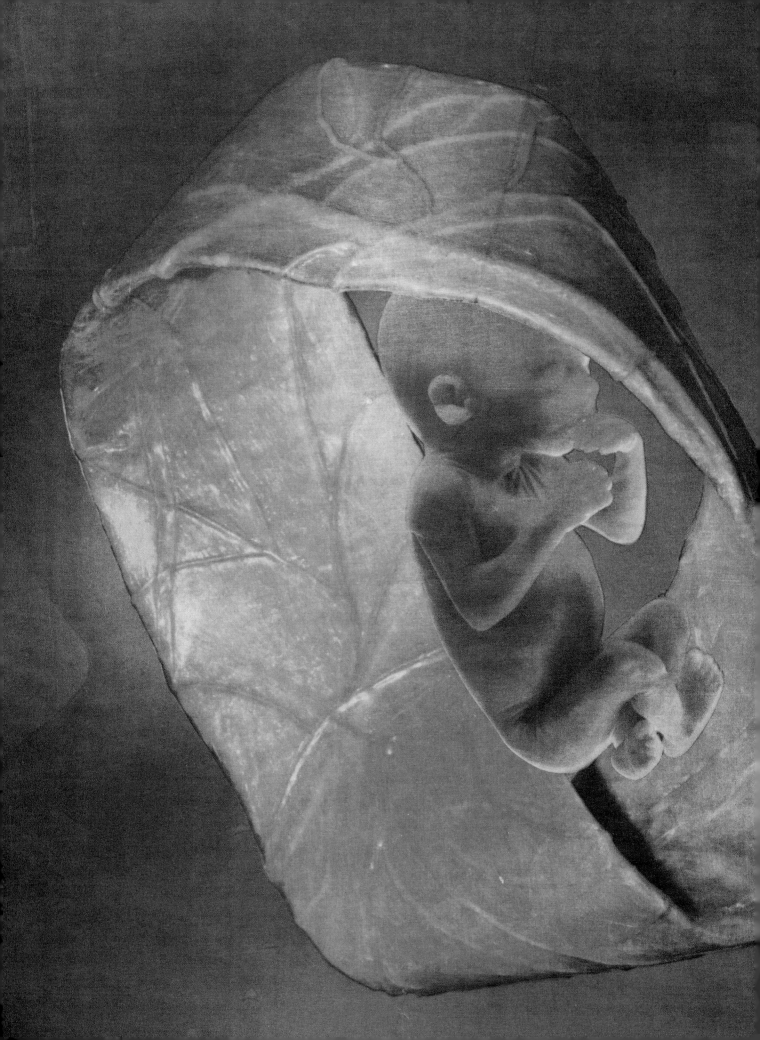

CHAPTER TWO

LIFE AFTER LIFE

Throughout history, many people have believed that their present life is only one of several. When they die, they expect to be reborn in a different form — reincarnated as another person, plant, or creature.

Humankind has always attempted to make sense of death by viewing it as a part of life — a new beginning, rather than an end. Belief in reincarnation is found in cultures throughout the world.

According to many anthropologists, humans have believed in reincarnation since early times. Although researchers can only speculate when there are no written records, burial practices and other customs often provide strong clues about the beliefs of ancient peoples. Many Stone Age graves, for example, contain bodies buried in the fetal position, perhaps in preparation for rebirth in a next life. Some people believed that the dead were reborn into their own families. Among Australian aborigines, newborn babies were shown to the tribal diviner in order to discover which deceased member of the tribe they had been in an earlier life.

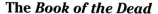

The Celts were so sure of living again that they would lend money on the promise of repayment in a future life.

Many ancient European cultures believed that human souls could transmigrate into animals, birds, and plants, as well as into other men and women. Celtic peoples held that the immortal soul passed from body to body for all eternity. Irish warriors had no fear of death, for they knew that if they were struck down in battle it was only the end of one of their many lives. The Celts were so sure of living again that they would even lend money on the promise of assured repayment in a future life.

The *Book of the Dead*
Death played a very important part in Egyptian culture. The pharaohs prepared for their deaths throughout their lives, building huge stone tombs called pyramids in which their carefully mummified bodies could rest secure throughout all eternity.

But the Egyptians believed that after the death of the body, the soul moved on. Egyptian holy writings, called the *Book of the Dead,* contain magical incantations that were supposed to free the soul from the tomb and allow it to be incarnated again. It could appear as a lotus, a hawk, a heron, a sycamore, a lily, or even a phoenix — which is the traditional symbol of rebirth in many cultures. After 3,000 years, moving from species to species in this way, the soul would be able to achieve rebirth again in another human form.

Belief in reincarnation is most closely identified with the great religions of the East — Hinduism and Buddhism. But the

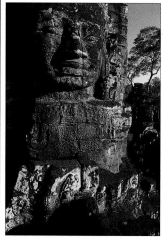

Carvings at Angkor Thom
A monument in celebration of Hinduism and Buddhism, the vast temple complex called the Bayon at Angkor Thom in Cambodia was built by the Khmer king Jayavarman VII in the 12th century. The stone is richly carved to represent the Hindu deities and demigods as well as the various incarnations of Buddha. The king believed himself to be the living Buddha, and so had himself depicted as many of these incarnations on the massive gates and towers.

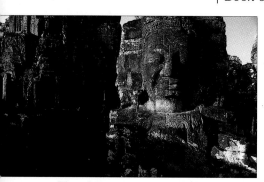

King Jayavarman as Buddha

Hindu religion was 3,000 years old before the concept became one of its fundamental tenets. Beginning about 1000 B.C., Hindu scriptures abound with colorful and detailed references to reincarnation. All souls are said to

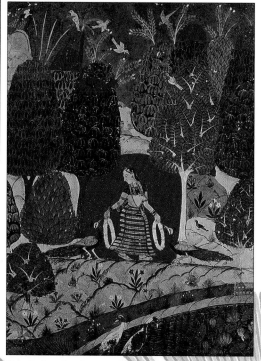

Symbols of reincarnation
Two peacocks stand on either side of a Mughal princess in this 18th-century Indian miniature. Peacocks are regarded as the bird of immortality and symbolize rebirth in Hinduism, Buddhism, and Islam. Until the 10th century A.D. they were also used in art to represent the figure of Christ himself.

emanate from an ultimate spiritual reality, to which they will return after many lives if they achieve spiritual purity. It is written in the *Upanishads*, ancient Hindu texts of around 650 B.C., that: "Those whose conduct here has been good will quickly attain a good birth as a Brahman or other superior caste. But those whose conduct has been evil will have an evil birth as a dog, a pig, or an untouchable outcast."

Hindus believe that we exist in a realm of illusion (called *maya*). Within this realm, souls are reincarnated across the whole spectrum of existence — animal, vegetable, even mineral. At death the soul returns to the Hindu heavens and is reborn in another form. It returns as a minor deity, human, or beast depending on whether goodness, passion, or darkness dominated in its

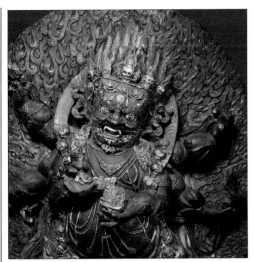

Reincarnation denied
This Tibetan image shows that 16th-century Buddhists believed that enemies of the faith would not achieve rebirth. The task of this grim-faced defender of the faith, or Dharmapalas, was to sever the roots of a nonbeliever's life with an ax, and then to collect the blood in a human skull.

previous existence. Only through spiritual progress made in its earthly lives can the soul develop beyond the cycle of reincarnation and reach the ultimate state of self-awareness and liberation (*moksha*).

Buddha, who lived about 500 years before Jesus Christ, was born a Hindu into the Brahman caste — the highest of the Indian castes. He claimed to have been through thousands of former lives

> "If I desire, I can by means of deva-vision ['god-sight'] recall all of my many former lives, up to ten, a thousand, a hundred thousand lives, or even more. I can give my experiences, both happy and unhappy, and all the circumstances and details, and the way my life ended."
>
> **Buddha**

(550 of which are described in a collection of tales called the *Jatakas*) before being incarnated as the Wise One and introducing Buddhism to the world. He taught that there is no personal self or soul, only a continuously changing, illusory ego, which keeps the wheel of rebirth moving. The endless cycle of rebirth comes to an end when the individual realizes that the personal self is a falsehood. This is *nirvana*, a condition of ultimate truth, blissful enlightenment, and freedom from desire.

Freedom of the soul
Rebirth theories also have an important, if less central place, in Western thought and theology. Many sophisticated thinkers of ancient Greece, beginning with the Orphics, a mystical sect of the 6th century B.C., believed in the idea of reincarnation. The Orphics viewed life as "the sorrowful weary wheel" from which the soul could escape by living a life of self-denial. The soul itself was seen as a separate, divine particle which was trapped in an earthly body from which it longed to be free. But freedom from this prison could be gained only after long ages of expiation and purification, as the soul passed through animal and human forms in a cycle of deaths and rebirths.

Members of other Greek sects were buried with notes directing the soul to ask for the pure water of remembrance so that they would recall their previous lives. For example, the Greek mathematician

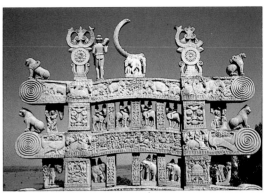

Buddhist stone carving
The north gate of the great Buddhist stupa, or shrine, at Sanchi, India, depicts myths relating to the Buddha's lives on earth in his previous human and animal incarnations.

Buddha entering nirvana
In this 18th-century Japanese painting, Shaka Muni (the Japanese name for Buddha) is shown entering nirvana, *the state of eternal bliss, as all creation mourns. Shaka Muni is a central figure of Zen Buddhism.*

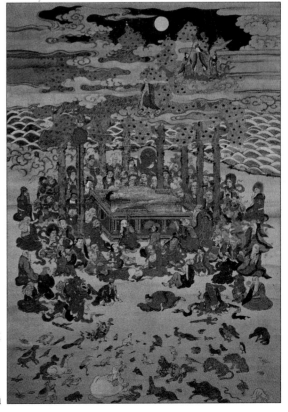

CYCLES OF REBIRTH

The Wheel of Life charts the soul's spiritual path through the physical world in life after life. This Tibetan Buddhist view of reincarnation — a central tenet of the faith — is frequently represented in temple paintings and carvings.

FOR BUDDHISTS, THE PHYSICAL WORLD that human beings experience as real, is mere illusion, part of the continuing cycle of birth, death, and rebirth known as *samsara*. Buddhists regard "self" as a misapprehension that traps humanity in the world. Once the conception of selfhood is shattered, the soul is freed from the imprisoning cycle of rebirth and attains *nirvana*, which is the state of perfect enlightenment.

Buddha, in the terrifying incarnation of Yama, the Lord of Death, holds the Wheel of Life. At the center of the wheel, three human motives — greed, hatred, and delusion — are represented in the form of three animals biting at each other's tails. Cutting through the sections of the main circle are the two paths the soul can take. To the right, the soul ascends toward the realm of the gods on the white path; to the left, the soul descends into the realm of infernal pain on the black path.

Realms of worldly existence

The third circle is divided into the six realms known as *lokas*. A person can be reborn in any *loka*. They consist of the realms of gods, titans, hungry ghosts, hell-beings, beasts, and humans.

On the right-hand side of the upper half is the realm of the gods. The beings living here have attained godly status through the good deeds performed in former lives, but they will be reborn in a lower realm. Buddhists are reminded that rebirth in heaven is not enough: they must strive for truth and wisdom. In the realm of infernal pain, the Judge of the Dead does not punish, but merely holds up the mirror of conscience, so that each soul can judge itself.

In the world of men, on the top left of the circle, human nature brings a chance to escape the rebirth cycle and to achieve *nirvana*. Diagonally opposite lies

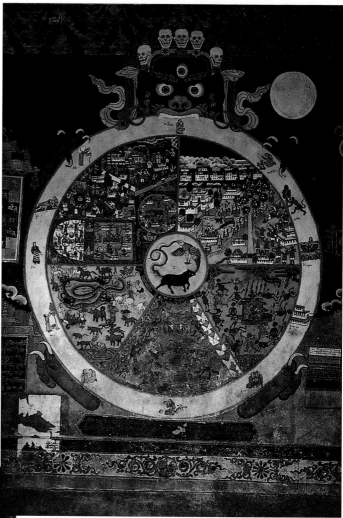

Buddhist wall painting
Beautiful examples of the symbolic Wheel of Life are a feature of virtually every Tibetan Buddhist temple.

the realm of hungry ghosts filled with unsatisfied passions causing endless human suffering. Buddha provides a release from the peaceless existence in the realm of the hungry ghosts. He carries the precious food that will satisfy the soul's cravings. This food is the desire for truth and knowledge that frees the soul from the illusion of the world.

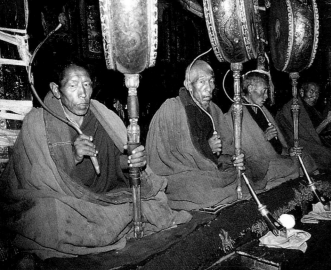

Lamas at evening prayer
The transmigration of the soul is central to the Tibetan Buddhist view of existence. Believers think that through spiritual exercise it is possible to free oneself from the cycle of reincarnation.

Pythagoras (*c.* 500 B.C.) claimed to have been a prophet, a fisherman, and even a prostitute, a peasant, and a shopkeeper's wife. The philosopher Xenophanes of Colphon satirized the idea of rebirth by claiming that he had asked a man to stop beating his dog, for he could recognize the voice of a dead friend in the dog's miserable howling. Others of the same period, such as the lyric poet Pindar and the philosopher Plato, also believed in reincarnation.

For Plato, souls were the very thread of life. At the moment of death, they chose a new life. Wise souls chose well but others were likely to make the wrong choice. Souls were born into one of nine states of probation — one of the highest being the philosopher. The souls expended energy in creating bodies for their new lives, and eventually, when the energy was exhausted, the soul disappeared. According to Plato, reincarnation is not an endless cycle.

Paying the price of a sinful life

The Romans also believed in reincarnation. The poet Virgil (70-19 B.C.) wrote about the souls of the dead drinking from Lethe, the river of forgetfulness that flowed through the underworld. They did this in order to forget their former lives before taking on new flesh. Sallust, a politician and historian who was a contemporary of Virgil, thought that the ills of the flesh proved the theory of reincarnation. Why else, Sallust maintained, should babies who have harmed no one be born blind or malformed? He believed that such seemingly unjust handicaps were a punishment for the evils of a former life. The early fathers of the Christian

Church, such as Origen, St. Augustine, and St. Jerome, perhaps influenced by Roman ideas, all believed in theories of reincarnation. Zoroastrianism, Mithraism, Manichaeism, and other cults popular in the Middle East during the second and third centuries A.D., all included reincarnation in their teachings. Some early Christians believed that souls were created blameless and would, after being purified in successive lives, finally enter heaven again in their original perfection. The idea of rebirth was grasped hopefully as it gave the soul more than one chance for salvation. But reincarnation never became part of orthodox Christian thought mainly because it cannot be reconciled with Christ's death on the cross. The New Testament makes it clear that each soul has only one life: "...it is appointed for men to die once, and after that comes judgment." (Hebrews 9:27).

The Judaic tradition on which Christianity rests also rejects reincarnation, although, in the Middle Ages, devotees of the Jewish mystical tradition known as the Cabala accepted the concept. In Jewish folklore the dybbuk, or evil spirit, is said to be a soul that remains wicked after three incarnations.

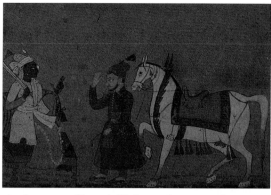

Vishnu reborn as a horse
One of the principal gods of Hinduism, Vishnu appears as the savior of mankind in 10 incarnations, or avatars. He is most famous as Lord Krishna, the divine shepherd. Vishnu also appears reincarnated as animals, such as the boar, horse, and fish. In this miniature Vishnu appears in his 10th reincarnation as the white horse, Kalki.

> # "It is appointed for men to die once, and after that comes judgment."
> ### (Hebrews 9:27)

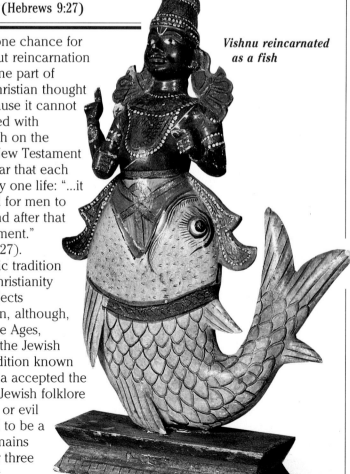

Vishnu reincarnated as a fish

Buddhist temple decoration
This 17th-century circular design appears on the Temple of the Tooth at Kandy in Sri Lanka.

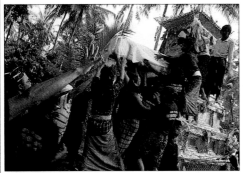

Balinese cremation
In Bali, Indonesia, two cremations are necessary — one for the body, the other for the soul. At the first cremation, the body is burned. The second cremation burns the soul, to free it for reincarnation.

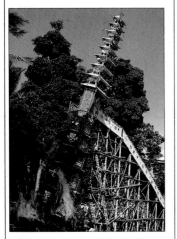

Cremating a soul in Bali

The ghats at Varanasi
At Varanasi in northern India, stone steps, known as ghats, lead down to the River Ganges. For Hindus, being cremated here breaks the karmic cycle of death and rebirth, freeing the soul.

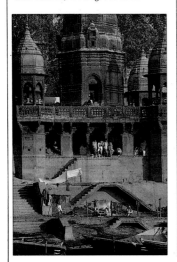

Many of the early Christian heresies involved belief in reincarnation. Even in the Middle Ages many people still held the idea, contrary to doctrine, that they would be reborn on earth. The heretical sects that taught rebirth were known collectively as Cathari. (Paradoxically, this name comes from the Greek word *katharoi* meaning "pure," and originates from St. Augustine's fourth-century writings on the Manichaeans, a religious sect to which he belonged.) Among the most famous of these heretical Cathari sects

---

Some modern Christians are able to reconcile a belief in some form of rebirth with their basic religious faith.

---

were the Albigensians, whose name derived from the city of Albi in southwestern France. The Albigensians flourished in the early 13th century, but in 1244 they paid the ultimate price for going against standard Catholic doctrine. The Albigensian retreat in the Pyrenees mountains, the castle of Montségur, was stormed by a group of crusading French barons. The heretics were all dragged out and executed.

A belief in reincarnation has no place among the official doctrines of the main Christian denominations, in which the afterlife consists of heaven, hell, purgatory, or limbo. However, some modern Christians are able to reconcile a belief in some form of rebirth with their basic religious faith.

In 1982, Geddes McGregor, Professor of Philosophy at the University of Southern California, published a book called *Reincarnation as a Christian Hope*, in which he suggested that reincarnation is an interpretation of the state of purgatory. Like McGregor, a growing number of thinkers from within the Western tradition are being influenced by Eastern religious concepts such as reincarnation.

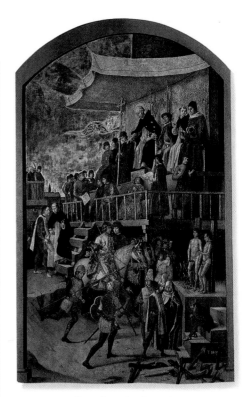

Burning the heretics
"St. Dominic Presides over the Burning of Heretics" is a 15th-century painting by the Spaniard Pedro Berruguete. St. Dominic founded the Dominican order to convert the Albigensian heretics, who believed in reincarnation.

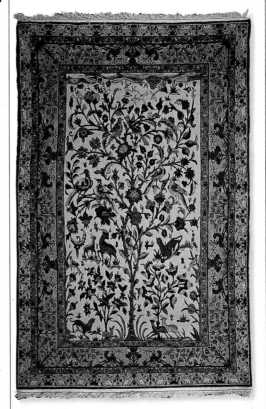

The tree of life
The tree of life motif on this Persian carpet symbolizes the relationship between the three worlds of the Islamic system of beliefs — paradise above, the world of men on earth, and hell below.

THE DALAI LAMA

The 14th dalai lama is the spiritual leader of millions of Tibetan Buddhists, all believers in reincarnation. They believe that the dalai lama is the embodiment of Chenrezi, the Buddhist god of grace, and that he has been returning to earth in different incarnations since 1391. On the death of one mortal body, he chooses a new one — and his followers begin the search to find the infant he has become.

THE SEARCH FOR the dalai lama ("greatest teacher") is undertaken by groups of lamas ("teachers") and monks using all the clues afforded by mystical tools such as the stars, visions, omens, and dreams. The dalai lama himself may have given hints before his death about where he has chosen to be reborn. The 13th dalai lama, who died in 1933, was said to have given a clue after his death. He was observed to have moved his head away from its original position, and toward the northeast. A star-shaped fungus then grew on the northeast side of the room housing the dalai lama's mausoleum, and a dragon flower appeared on the northeast side of the main courtyard. The high lamas were convinced that the child they sought would be found in that direction.

A sacred quest

The lamas had another clue. A high ranking monk had had a vision of the future at the Lake of Chos Khorgyal, a sacred Buddhist site. In it he glimpsed a distinctive house with carved gables and blue eaves. The lamas knew that they had only to find this house, and the child would be nearby. In 1937 the lamas set off to the northeast, and traveled for two years, going deep into Chinese territory, before they found the vital sign. When they reached a village called Takster they saw a house with carved gables and blue eaves. They knew that they were near the end of their quest.

Donning the robes of a servant to hide his senior rank, one of the high lamas entered the house with the blue eaves. There, a two-year-old boy called Tenzin Gyatso demanded the rosary from around the disguised monk's neck. It had been the dalai lama's. The child then correctly identified other items — rosaries, a drum, a walking stick — that had belonged to the dalai lama. For the searching lamas, Gyatso's

true identity was confirmed by physical signs (large ears, and moles and birthmarks) that are found on the body of every dalai lama. The boy and his family were brought back to Tibet so that the child could begin the rigorous course of study that would enable him to lead the Tibetan nation. But first the monks had to pay a ransom demanded by the Chinese governor of the province: 300,000 Chinese yuan (about $300,000) for the child's freedom.

The process of searching for a reborn spirit is also carried out when a more ordinary lama dies. Lama Yeshe, a Tibetan Buddhist whose spiritual mission had been to bring Buddhism to the West, died in 1984. Eleven months after his death, a couple in a tiny

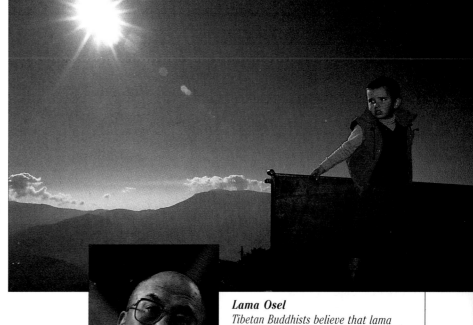

Lama Osel
Tibetan Buddhists believe that lama Yeshe was reincarnated as Osel Hita Torres, born near Granada, Spain.

The present dalai lama
It took a search party of high lamas two years to track down the present incarnation of the dalai lama, in a small village in China.

mountain village near Granada, Spain, had their fifth child, Osel Hita Torres. The couple, who were devout Buddhists and who had built a meditation center in the mountains outside Granada, had been known to lama Yeshe during his lifetime. Osel was revealed as the reborn lama after undergoing the traditional tests identifying items belonging to lama Yeshe.

Lama Osel was enthroned in March 1987 in an ancient ceremony high in the mountains of northern India. For Tibetan Buddhists, this was the final proof that lama Yeshe had returned — reincarnated in the person of a young Spanish boy.

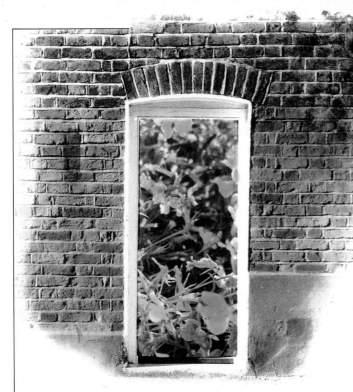

CASEBOOK

Going Back to Mom's House

"Where did this girl get all this information?"

As soon as toddler Romy Crees began to speak in the early 1980's, she kept talking about wanting to go home. As her verbal skills improved, she also began to tell stories of her own death in a motorcycle accident. "I'm afraid of motorcycles," she said.

Romy, who lived with her family in Des Moines, Iowa, described where she grew up: "I lived in a red brick house and went to school in Charles City." Charles City is about 120 miles northeast of Des Moines. Romy said her name was Joe Williams, she was married to Sheila, and they had three children. Romy also said "Mother Williams' name is Louise, and she has a pain in her right leg."

Preoccupation with the past

As Romy continued to tell stories about her previous life, her parents began seriously to consider the possibility of reincarnation. They decided to contact Hemendra Banerjee, a well-known researcher into extracerebral memory who had been featured in several newspaper articles and appeared on television.

Banerjee was the founder of the Indian Institute of Parapsychology, and he had moved to Los Angeles in 1970. Romy's continued preoccupation with the life of Joe Williams eventually persuaded Banerjee and the family that a trip to Charles City was in order.

Accompanied by some journalists, the group set off for Charles City. Romy told her parents that when they arrived at the house they wouldn't be able to go in the front door, but would have to use the back door. She also said that she wanted to buy some blue flowers.

When they arrived at the town, Romy was unsure of the address of the Williams home. One of the group checked in the telephone book and noted the address of a Louise Williams. When they pulled up in front of the house, it was a white bungalow, not a red brick house as they had been led to believe. However, there was a sign at the front door asking visitors to go round the back. When Louise Williams answered the door, she moved very slowly because of the severe pain in her right leg. She did not want to be disturbed because she was on her way to the doctor's office, but said they could come back later.

Gift of remembrance

Later, when they returned, Mrs. Williams unwrapped the bouquet of flowers. She was surprised at the choice of flowers because the last gift her son had given her before his fatal motorcycle accident was a bunch of blue flowers. While they were talking, Mrs. Williams said that her family had lived in a red brick house, but it had been destroyed by a tornado that had damaged a great deal of Charles City 10 years earlier, in 1971.

Louise could not believe what she heard when the Crees related Romy's memories of the Williams household. Louise said, "Where did this girl get all this information?" Romy and Mrs. Williams went into another room of the house. When they returned, Mrs. Williams said that Romy had managed to identify all of the members of Joe's family and several other people from photographs that had been on display in the room. "She recognized them!" Louise said with a sense of amazed disbelief, "She actually recognized them!"

My Sister Is Back

Susan's unexplained knowledge was "harmonious...with the interpretation that Susan somehow had access to Winnie's memories."

THE EASTLAND FAMILY from Idaho suffered a terrible loss when their six-year-old daughter Winnie was killed by a passing car in 1961. About six months after Winnie's death, her sister Sharon dreamed that Winnie was going to return to the family. She had no idea how this would happen, but she was convinced it was true. After another two years, Mrs. Eastland became pregnant. Mr. Eastland reported hearing a voice telling him that Winnie would be rejoining them. Although the family still thought a great deal about Winnie, they were very skeptical about any possible reincarnation.

Family likeness
When Susan was born, she was a delight to the whole family. After she began to speak, Susan consistently said that she was six years old. The bubbly little girl also showed an unusual interest in two photos of Winnie and insisted they were pictures of her, not the deceased sister she never knew. Little Susan also seemed to have an unusual and unaccountable knowledge of Winnie. Although Susan never referred to herself as Winnie, she often used to scribble Winnie's name on pieces of paper.

Susan knew the game
While Winnie was alive, the family used to play a little game with the cookie jar. The lid of the cookie container was in the shape of a cat. When the children wanted a cookie, they had to ask the cat. Mrs. Eastland would then answer as if she were the cat and tell them how many cookies they were allowed to have. Not long after Winnie died, Mrs. Eastland wrapped up the cookie jar and stored it away. A few years later she came across it and decided to use it again. To her complete surprise, Susan knew all about the game of asking the cat for cookies, and even mimicked her mother's

high-pitched version of the cat's response. Susan also told her mother about an incident she remembered when they were at the local bowling alley. She said that while she was playing near the food and candy counters, she had been kissed by a boy. This incident certainly had happened to Winnie and had not been forgotten by her family. Mr. Eastland in particular had been very annoyed when he had heard about it and had not wanted it mentioned ever again.

Mysterious memories
Psychiatrist Dr. Ian Stevenson, a leading researcher on reincarnation, studied the case of Susan Eastland. After his conversations with her he stated that Susan's unexplained knowledge was "harmonious...with the interpretation that Susan somehow had access to Winnie's memories." The evidence of paranormal knowledge could not be considered conclusive, but Susan's knowledge of Winnie's life was too detailed to be explained by contact with the rest of the family.

HYPNOTIC MEMORIES

Startling evidence to support the theory of reincarnation has come from subjects under hypnosis talking about what happened in their past lives.

THE SPANIARD FERNANDO COLAVIDA was one of the first hypnotists to attempt age regression in 1887. This technique takes a subject back in time to, say, his or her seventh birthday. By means of hypermnesia (the ability to tap memory to an abnormal extent), every detail of the birthday is recalled.

The technique proved useful in discovering the causes of phobias and neuroses. Some hypnotists regressed their subjects to very early experiences, including those undergone at birth or in the womb. The next step was to inquire into experiences that happened even before conception. It was then discovered that some people, under hypnosis, claimed to have lived before, and could give detailed and fascinating accounts of these lives.

Some consider Dr. Mortis Stark to have pioneered the use of hypnosis to regress subjects to past lives in 1906. However, in 1911 a Frenchman, Albert de Rochas, published an account of experiments that probably took place before much of Dr. Stark's work.

The case of Bridey Murphy

Popular interest in past-life remembrances was rekindled in the late 1950's following the publication of Dr. Morey Bernstein's book, *The Search for Bridey Murphy*. The Bridey Murphy case was fiercely debated in the press and subsequently made into a film.

Bernstein was an accomplished amateur hypnotist. His subject was 29-year-old Virginia Burns Tighe from Madison, Wisconsin. The hypnotic sessions began in November 1952 and lasted nearly a year. Under hypnosis Mrs. Tighe revealed that in a previous life she had been an Irish girl named Bridey Murphy.

Bridey was described as having been born on December 20, 1798, into a Protestant family living in Cork. She married a Catholic by the name of Brian Joseph McCarthy, and traveled with him to Belfast, where she lived until her death in 1864. Bridey supposedly died by falling downstairs, breaking her hip.

The drabness of Bridey's life as described by Virginia Burns Tighe is typical of many revealed under hypnosis. Contrary to popular belief, comparatively few subjects claim to have been such

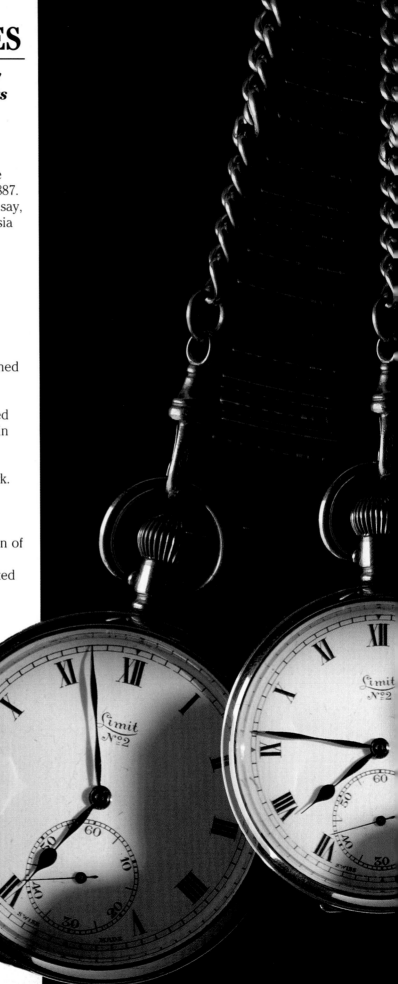

♦ PAGE 53

A STATE OF TRANCE

For many people, the idea of being put into a hypnotic trance is a little sinister. In reality, the whole process is quite straightforward:

◆ The subject is made comfortable. An object, such as a pencil or watch, is held about 12 inches away and the subject is asked to concentrate upon it.

◆ The hypnotist makes a series of suggestions over and over again in a monotonous tone, introducing the idea of relaxation, followed by drowsiness, heaviness, warmth, and, finally, sleep.

◆ The hypnotist can then make a further series of suggestions from which the depth of the trance can be measured. He may suggest that an arm has become very heavy and see if the subject can lift it.

◆ Traditional methods simply involved the patient responding to the hypnotist's questions. Modern therapists encourage subjects to expand their answers on their own initiative.

◆ In order to "awaken" the subject at the end of the session, the hypnotist will help him or her to leave the hypnotic state gradually, usually by counting.

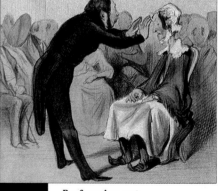

Performing art
In the 19th century, hypnotism became popular as an entertainment. This caricature shows the celebrated French hypnotist Robert Macaire at work.

HIDDEN EVIDENCE

One very plausible explanation for the phenomenon of past lives discovered through hypnotic regression is that of cryptomnesia. Subconscious memories surface during hypnosis, surprising both subject and hypnotist, and often appearing in the guise of a past life.

IN 1969 IN CARDIFF, WALES, hypnotherapist Arnall Bloxham regressed "Jane Evans" to six previous lives: as Livonia (wife of Titus, tutor to the young Constantine, future emperor of Rome) living in York in the fourth century A.D.; then as Rebecca, a Jewish woman, massacred in York in 1190; third, as Alison, who died in 1451, the teenage servant of a French merchant prince, Jacques Coeur; fourth, as Anna, servant to Catherine of Aragon (1485-1536); fifth, as Ann Tasker, a London servant girl in Queen Anne's reign (*c*.1700); finally as Sister Grace, née Ellis, an American nun who died in about 1920. Prof. Brian Hartley, an expert on Roman Britain, commented that the events of the first life were mostly correct, and some of the knowledge was "quite remarkable."

The most dramatic life was that of Rebecca, whose personality was entirely different from that of Jane. She said that she died in a massacre of Jewish people in 1190 in the crypt of St. Mary's, Castlegate. This church was not known to have a crypt – but one was discovered (though dating from well after 1190) after

Jane was plainly terrified as she recalled the violent mob entering the crypt.

"Rebecca" had revealed its existence. Although the massacre of the Jews of York was a real historical event, it occurred in the keep of York Castle, not in St. Mary's crypt. However, Jane was plainly terrified as she recalled the mob entering the crypt. Only a superb actress could have simulated such a state of mind.

Inspired by works of fiction

Not surprisingly, Jane's case aroused public interest. Much detective work was done by the media to try to authenticate the "past lives." As a result of the investigations, particularly those carried out by writer and broadcaster Melvin Harris, the real sources of Jane Evans's past lives have been discovered. "Livonia" had her origins in a book by Louis de Wohl called *The Living Wood*. Under hypnosis, Jane Evans returned to

fourth-century Britain and recalled her life as Livonia – but all her "memories" can be traced to the book. For example, Wohl's fictional characters Curio and Valerius appear as real people in the "past life." Jane Evans's other lives were also inspired by works of fiction: most of her memories came directly from books she had read. It seems likely that "Rebecca" had

Her regression accounts were not of previous existences, but came from somewhere deep in her subconscious.

her first incarnation in a BBC radio play; teenage servant "Alison" originated in *The Moneyman* by T. B. Costain; Catherine of Aragon's servant "Anna" apparently came from a Jean Plaidy novel, *Katherine, The Virgin Widow*.

There was never any suggestion that Jane Evans was a conscious fraud. But it appeared that her regression accounts were not in fact of previous existences, but came from somewhere deep in her subconscious. In this case, the proof of cryptomnesia was conclusive. Evans's "hidden memory" of particular fictional works surfaced in the accounts she gave to hypnotherapist Arnall Bloxham. This case shows how careful researchers must be in drawing conclusions from evidence obtained under hypnosis.

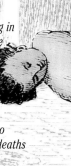

Massacre at York
During anti-Semitic rioting in York, England, in 1190, the city's Jews took shelter in York Castle. When the keep was stormed, many Jews killed their children and themselves to avoid savage and brutal deaths at the hands of the mob.

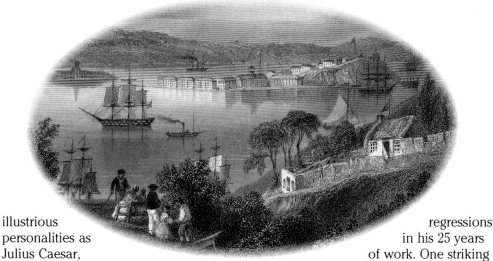

The Cove of Cork, Ireland

illustrious personalities as Julius Caesar, Abraham Lincoln, or Napoleon. Mrs. Tighe's case was thoroughly investigated. A number of extremely obscure facts that she could not have known from normal sources were proved accurate. For example, she described a contemporary method of kissing the Blarney Stone that was different from the modern way. Other details, however, were not correct, and many others could not be confirmed. Tighe had never been to Ireland. However, there were allegations, which she denied, that she had been familiar with a number of Irish people in her youth.

Ultimately it was never possible to confirm whether Bridey Murphy had ever existed. But in the controversy over Mrs. Tighe's regression, the advantage seemed to lie with those who held that it was genuine. Fraud appeared to be impossible because of the obscurity of the material. The correctness of some details was discovered only by research in Ireland, and this information would certainly have been inaccessible to most Americans, including Mrs. Tighe.

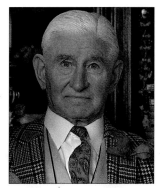

Dr. Morey Bernstein and Virginia Tighe

Stress under hypnosis

The Bridey Murphy case is probably the most widely known, but there are many others. Spiritualist Alexander Cannon, working in the 1950's, was convinced of reincarnation by the 1,382 hypnotic sessions he conducted. In *Encounters with the Past* (1979) hypnotherapist Joe Keeton records facilitating 800 regressions in his 25 years of work. One striking Keeton case was the regression of "Jan." Under hypnosis this young woman became 18-year-old Joan Waterhouse, tried for witchcraft at the Chelmsford Assizes in 1566. Not only was nearly every detail historically correct, but "Joan" showed all the emotional stress expected of a girl on trial for her life.

In 1976 Arnall Bloxham, a Welsh hypnotherapist, became well known to British television audiences after the showing of a BBC documentary *The Bloxham Tapes*. During the course of his work, Bloxham regressed over 400 subjects into past lives.

A particularly striking Bloxham regression was that of Graham Huxtable, who changed from being a charming, soft-spoken Welshman to a "swearing, illiterate gunner's mate," serving in the Royal Navy in the Napoleonic wars. An intriguing aspect of this case was that Huxtable used archaic naval slang and made references to shipboard practices that were typical of this period. These practices were confirmed as accurate by National Maritime Museum historians. The sailor's piercing screams of agony when his leg was shot off in battle show either the reliving of an actual experience or an outstanding acting ability.

POSSIBLE EXPLANATIONS

It has so far been impossible to prove the authenticity of past-life regressions such as those obtained by Arnall Bloxham and others through hypnosis. But research has produced an interesting variety of possible explanations for the phenomenon.

Cryptomnesia

Under hypnosis some subjects are able to recall minute details of books, films, or events they experienced years before and only for a split second. This hidden memory suggests the existence of mental resources so far untapped.

The mythopoeic faculty

In certain altered states of consciousness, people have been known to develop incredible talents, such as the ability to paint, sing, or compose. This faculty, if applied to acting ability, could explain the amazing theatrical "performances" of some regression subjects.

Extrasensory perception

This paranormal solution is hard to accept and almost impossible to prove. But in theory no historical detail, no matter how long ago it was recorded, could escape the probings of a mind made open to ESP through the process of hypnosis.

Multiple personalities

A second life that surfaces during a hypnotic regression may not be a past life at all, but the expression of a second, separate, personality existing in the present. In such cases it is vital that the subject seek further professional help and guidance.

Another time, another place
Arnall Bloxham has explored the strange world of people whose memories of previous lives suggest they may have been reincarnated.

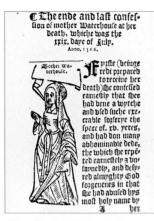

The Chelmsford witches
The original pamphlet describing the trial of Joan Waterhouse and her mother gives the date correctly as 1566. An edition published in the 19th century contains a crucial misprint, giving the date of the trial as 1556. The fact that Joe Keeton's subject supplied the wrong date, 1556, proves that her information came from the 19th-century pamphlet and not from the event itself.

THE EXAMINA-
tion and confeſſion of cer-
taine Wytches at Chenſforde in
the Countie of Eſſex before
the Quenes maieſties
Judges, the XXVI
daye of July
Anno 1556

At the Aſſiſe holden there
as then, and one of them
put to death for the ſame
offence, as their examination declareth more
at large.

The 19th-century reprint

Regression experiences such as those reported by Bernstein, Cannon, Keeton, and Bloxham seem to present a watertight case for reincarnation. There are, however, other possible explanations, including cryptomnesia, the mythopoeic faculty, ESP, and multiple personalities.

Walking encyclopedias
Psychological studies have revealed that our subconscious memories are far more extensive than our conscious recall. Much of the subconscious can be tapped only by techniques such as hypnosis. Some psychologists maintain that we subconsciously remember everything we experience. For example, it is possible to thumb casually through the pages of a book without consciously absorbing more than an odd sentence. Years later, under hypnosis, we may reproduce accurately whole pages, punctuation and all. Such cryptomnesia (hidden memory) appears to be miraculous, but its existence has been demonstrated beyond doubt.

Every day we are bombarded with information from newspapers, television and radio, books and magazines. If it is true that it all remains "on file," we are full of more miscellaneous data than any encyclopedia. We cannot say for certain that the most obscure fact, ostensibly produced as part of a former life, has not been picked up from some source forgotten by the conscious mind.

The mythopoeic faculty is the ability possessed by some, perhaps all, human beings to show talent far beyond conscious powers when in a state of dissociation (a condition in which certain mental processes operate independently of the normal state of waking consciousness). Thus subjects may sketch in the style of old masters, or produce music in the manner of great composers. More to the point, they may even act the parts of former life personalities as well as any professional actor. The combination of cryptomnesia and the mythopoeic faculty may be enough to explain the phenomenon of past lives discovered by hypnotic regression.

It is argued, however, that facts so obscure that they are proved accurate only by intense research can never have come to the attention of ordinary people. The paranormal theory of extrasensory perception (ESP) is one way of explaining this detailed knowledge. ESP is the acquisition of information outside our usual sensory and mental powers.

Some psychics believe that it is possible to use ESP to tap into an ultimate information source, known as the Akashic Records (from the Sanskrit *akasha*, meaning the fundamental substance of the universe). Famous healer and psychic Edgar Cayce stated that these records exist on the universe's spiritual plane as a register of everything thought, said, and done in the history of humankind. A person with access to such limitless material could reveal details of countless lives during hypnotic regression, without having actually experienced any of them.

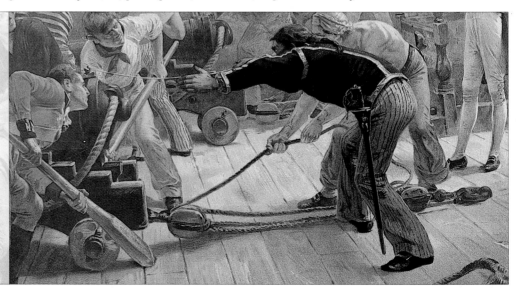

A sailor's life
One of Bloxham's subjects recounted a past life as a gunner's mate in the Royal Navy during the time of Admiral Lord Nelson. This was a glorious but gory period in naval history, and the session culminated in the sailor having his leg shot off by a cannonball.

It's not necessary to look for farfetched theories, such as the Akashic Records, to explain the detailed knowledge often revealed in regression cases. Sometimes it is easy to demonstrate how ordinary people pick up obscure facts. The one important incorrect detail in the Joan Waterhouse regression already mentioned is pointed out by the historian Ian Wilson in his book *Mind Out of Time*. Joan insisted that she was tried in Elizabeth I's reign in 1556, but it was actually Queen Mary who was on the throne at that time. In reality the trial took place 10 years later in 1566. An account of the event appeared in a pamphlet of which only one copy survives, in Lambeth Palace Library,

between lives are often inconsistent and reflect either the culture of the subjects or the outlook of the hypnotist. Albert de Rochas's subjects, mainly Catholics, see their dead bodies protected from devils by the priestly sprinklings of holy water, while Alexander Cannon's dead spirits are shepherded by "white brothers" and a "blue sister" in a spiritualist garden. It may be that suggestible subjects simply do not want to disappoint the hypnotist, and that the mere mention of regression before they go under may prompt them to create a suitably interesting life or series of lives.

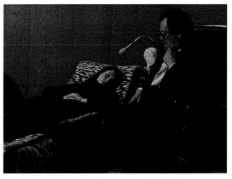

A hypnotherapy session

REGRESSION THERAPY

Events occurring early in life may inspire such terror or guilt that those who experience them refuse to face them. Such a memory is consequently pushed into the subconscious. Here it remains hidden and can fester, resulting in phobias or neuroses that may need psychiatric help in later life. One type of treatment uses techniques, including hypnosis, that help the patient to remember and face the hidden terror, which is usually not as appalling as it seemed to be when it happened.

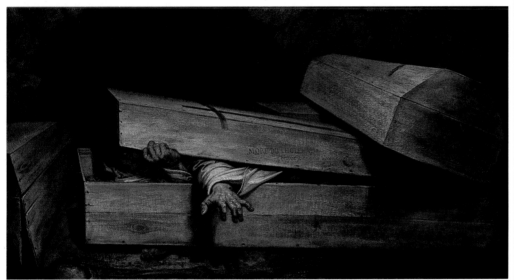

Buried alive

This 19th-century Belgian painting by Antoine Wiertz explores the horror of premature burial. Such an event has been suggested as a cause of severe claustrophobia in a subsequent life.

London — a place Jane had never visited. In the 19th century the British Philobiblon Society, specialists in reproducing limited editions of very rare books, reissued the pamphlet and the printer mistakenly set the date on the title page as 1556, an error later repeated by several writers. The mistake proves that the facts Jane was remembering came from written material, not from personal experience.

Factual corroboration

Hypnotically produced previous incarnations have revealed some striking former existences in exotic places such as Atlantis or ancient Egypt. However, in such cases subjects rarely use a former language or give any description of local customs. In addition, the experiences of hypnotized subjects in the intermission

Consequently, most researchers into reincarnation experiences regard material discovered using hypnotic regression as flawed.

Nevertheless, it is difficult to be entirely disbelieving when a personality changes several times, or a subject "dies" convincingly in the chair as he or she is brought to the end of a previous life. Extensive research is often needed to confirm the details thrown out so casually by the subject, so a conscious attempt at deception seems unlikely. But the precise mechanism by which this extraordinary phenomenon is produced still remains a compelling mystery.

Phobias from past lives

Medical hypnotists normally investigate only present-day memories. Reincarnationists, such as Roger Woolger in the U.S. and Dr. Denys Kelsey in Britain, believe that phobias may be caused by terrifying experiences in former existences. For example, acute fear of water could indicate that a previous life had ended by drowning. Extreme claustrophobia might derive from the subject's suffocation in a coffin after being buried while in a coma, mistaken for dead.

A shadow in the water

Medical records report the case of a girl who was competing in a diving contest and was suddenly stricken with panic by the sight of a shadow moving in the water. Under hypnosis, she appeared to return to a past life that ended with her seeing a similar shadow as she jumped into water. The girl was convinced that the shadow was that of an alligator that had attacked and killed her in a previous life.

FAMOUS BELIEVERS

Many well-known people — including such scientific figures as Henry Ford — have professed a profound belief in some kind of reincarnation after this life.

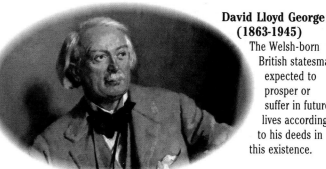

David Lloyd George (1863-1945)
The Welsh-born British statesman expected to prosper or suffer in future lives according to his deeds in this existence.

THE 16TH-CENTURY ITALIAN philosopher Giordano Bruno taught that a soul passed from one body to another and could ultimately attain perfection. Bruno paid painfully for his views, being burned at the stake as a heretic. A century later, Voltaire affirmed reincarnation to be "neither absurd nor useless....It is no more surprising to be born twice than to be born once...everything in nature is resurrection." The German philosopher Immanuel Kant believed that souls existed prior to earthly life and that they traveled to other planets after inhabiting human bodies. Johann Wolfgang von Goethe supported the philosophers. "I am certain that I have been here, as I am now, a thousand times before," he wrote, "and I hope to return a thousand times."

Belief in reincarnation was shared in varying degrees by such prominent English poets as William Blake, Samuel Taylor Coleridge, William Wordsworth, and Percy Bysshe Shelley. For his part, Ralph Waldo Emerson was influenced by the *Bhagavadgita*, the Hindu holy work, and likened successive lives to climbing stairs. Walt Whitman and Herman Melville both believed in rebirth. Gustav Stromberg, the astronomer-physicist, wrote that the human soul,

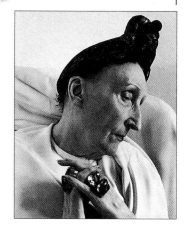

Dame Edith Sitwell (1887-1964)
The English poet often remarked on her striking facial resemblance to the Tudor English king Henry VII and his granddaughter, Queen Elizabeth I. Dame Edith suggested that she may have been Henry VII in a former life.

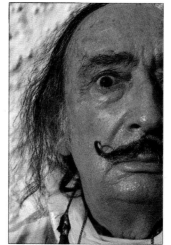

"indestructible and immortal, carries an indelible record of all its activities." Rider Haggard, the novelist, claimed to have been a Norseman, a Zulu, and an Egyptian in earlier lives. Carl Jung believed that "one's life is prolonged in time by passing through different bodily existences." This sentiment is one that composers Richard Wagner, Gustav Mahler, and Jean Sibelius have endorsed.

Salvador Dali (1904-89)
The surrealist painter considered himself to be a reincarnation of St. John of the Cross, the 16th-century Spanish mystic of the Carmelite Order.

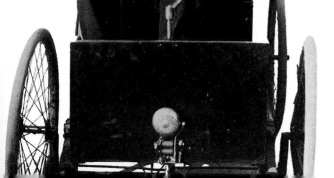

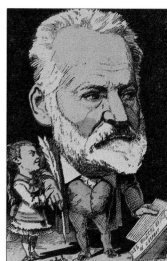

Victor Hugo (1802-85)
The French novelist wrote that when he died it would be as if he had merely finished a day's work — which he would resume the next morning.

Henry Ford (1863-1947)
The automotive inventor believed that genius, including his own, resulted from long experience gained in the course of many previous lives.

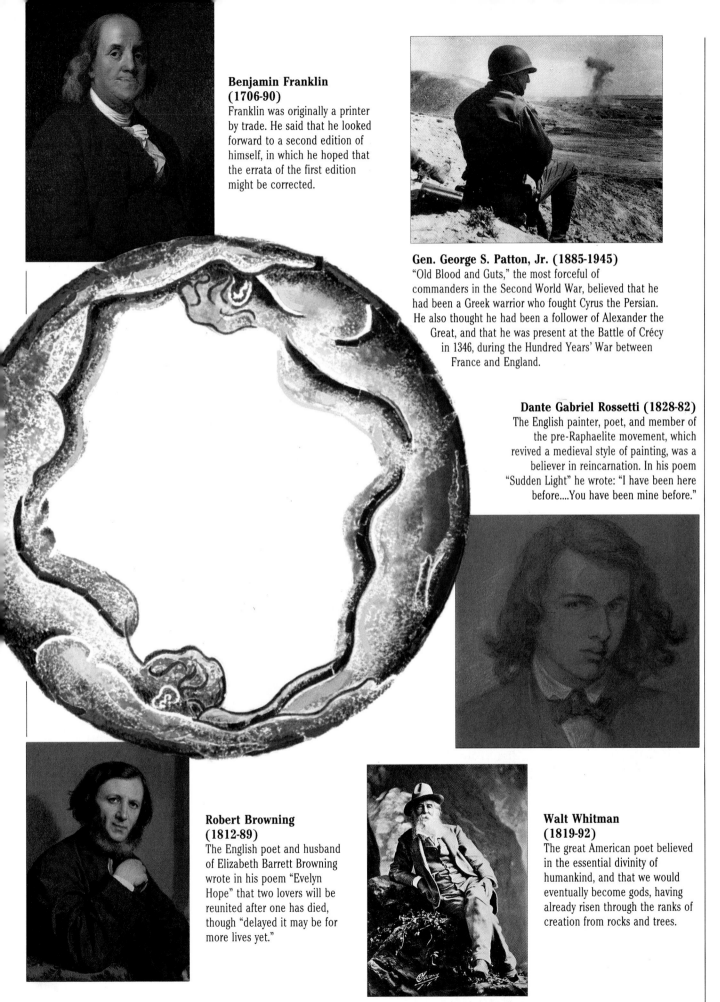

Benjamin Franklin (1706-90)
Franklin was originally a printer by trade. He said that he looked forward to a second edition of himself, in which he hoped that the errata of the first edition might be corrected.

Gen. George S. Patton, Jr. (1885-1945)
"Old Blood and Guts," the most forceful of commanders in the Second World War, believed that he had been a Greek warrior who fought Cyrus the Persian. He also thought he had been a follower of Alexander the Great, and that he was present at the Battle of Crécy in 1346, during the Hundred Years' War between France and England.

Dante Gabriel Rossetti (1828-82)
The English painter, poet, and member of the pre-Raphaelite movement, which revived a medieval style of painting, was a believer in reincarnation. In his poem "Sudden Light" he wrote: "I have been here before....You have been mine before."

Robert Browning (1812-89)
The English poet and husband of Elizabeth Barrett Browning wrote in his poem "Evelyn Hope" that two lovers will be reunited after one has died, though "delayed it may be for more lives yet."

Walt Whitman (1819-92)
The great American poet believed in the essential divinity of humankind, and that we would eventually become gods, having already risen through the ranks of creation from rocks and trees.

A PLACE, NOT A PERSON

Ginger, as Sarah Jean, described traveling on a riverboat ....and then went on to recount her suicide by drowning.

MANY PAST-LIFE MEMORIES seem to surface when the subject is very young, generally between the ages of two and five. In the case of the woman who was given the pseudonym Ginger Waldorf, the memories did not begin to manifest themselves until she was 20 years old. Ginger Waldorf was born in 1948 in a small town in Ohio. She was placed for adoption when she was four years old and was shunted between several foster homes after that. She was a shy, insecure child, and she grew up to be intensely religious.

Hazy recollections

After she was married, Ginger moved with her husband to Texas. The birth of their first child prompted Ginger to try to trace her own biological parents. She felt that she had a clue to her origins as the name Marietta had been coming into her mind for some time. She thought perhaps she had originally been called Marietta, or that it was the name of her natural mother.

Ginger decided to undergo a session of hypnotic regression to recall details of her early childhood and natural parents. She hoped that this might help in her search. While she was in the hypnotic state, it became clear that the name Marietta referred to the town in Ohio, not a person as Ginger had originally assumed. Thinking that Marietta might be the town where she had spent her early childhood, Ginger went there, and found at once that the area seemed completely familiar. This, thought Ginger, was certainly the place where she had spent her earliest years.

By tracking back through the foster homes of her childhood, Ginger finally contacted her natural mother and met some of her sisters. Surprisingly, they were not the least bit familiar with Marietta, Ohio, nor could they share the other memories that Ginger had recorded during the hypnotic sessions. For the first time, Ginger considered the possibility of reincarnation. After some deliberation, she decided to investigate the possibility further. Ginger consulted a psychologist, who referred her to the Psychical Research Foundation in Carrollton, Georgia.

Fear of water

After several hypnotic sessions probing into Ginger's memory, she recalled her name as Sarah Jean Jenkins and her address in Marietta. Ginger described the way the town looked in her former life at the turn of the century and recalled the names of several of her relatives. When these details of stores, buildings, and peoples' names were checked against public records, they matched perfectly. During one hypnotic session, Ginger, as Sarah Jean, described traveling on a riverboat. She recalled the name of the captain, and then went on to recount her suicide by drowning.

Ginger had always had an intense fear of water. Perhaps the fear was carried over from her past life as Sarah Jean Jenkins and the horrible way she died.

In the hypnotic sessions, Sarah Jean seemed to take over Ginger's personality completely. Both the voice of Sarah Jean and her extremely confident manner expressed a character totally different from Ginger's, and one that the diffident and insecure Ginger could only envy.

NOW THEY ARE TWINS

Jennifer picked up one of the dolls and said: "Oh, that's Mary and this is my Suzanne. I haven't seen her for such a long time."

THE DEATH OF THE TWO young Pollock sisters shattered the lives of their parents, John and Florence. John Pollock of Scarborough in northern England had always maintained a firm belief in reincarnation but it provided little consolation when the two girls were killed by a passing car as they made their way to Mass on the sunny morning of May 5, 1957. Joanna was 11 years old at the time while her younger sister Jacqueline was only six.

Certain knowledge

Eight months after the accident, Mrs. Pollock informed her husband that she was pregnant. Mr. Pollock was convinced that his wife would give birth to twins who would be the reincarnation of their two daughters. Mrs. Pollock refused to entertain any such idea. After a later examination at the gynecologist's, she was able to inform her husband that there was no chance of twins. The doctor stated that there was only one heartbeat evident and one set of limbs. To Mrs. Pollock, it seemed that any possibility of reincarnation of the two girls was finally confounded. Mr. Pollock was unshaken and insisted that he would be proved right.

Identical twins with a difference

When Mrs. Pollock went into labor on the night of October 3, 1958, the attending midwife said to Mr. Pollock: "I wish you'd accept that twins won't be born." Early the next morning, Mr. Pollock, who was a milkman, was making his rounds. He was told then that his wife had in fact given birth to identical twins.

When identical twins are born, they are expected to have identical birthmarks. In the case of the Pollock girls, Jennifer, who was born 10 minutes after Gillian, had a faint white line across her forehead which matched the scar that Jacqueline (the younger of the two dead sisters) had developed as a result of a fall when she was two years old. Jennifer also had the same brown thumbprint on her thigh that marked Jacqueline. Her sister, Gillian, had neither mark.

When the girls were toddlers, their father opened up a box of toys that had belonged to the two dead girls and that had been put away after the accident. When the twins saw the toys, Jennifer picked up one of the dolls and said: "Oh, that's Mary and this is my Suzanne.

I haven't seen her for such a long time." Mr. Pollock found an old smock that his wife used to wear to meet the girls from school. When Jennifer saw the smock, she said: "That's what mummy wore when she fetched us from school." Mrs. Pollock had not worn the smock since the deaths of Joanna and Jacqueline. In 1966 Indian researcher Hemendra Banerjee interviewed the Pollock sisters. The case was reported widely in the national press and helped to establish Banerjee as a leading investigator into reincarnation.

Several other incidents have supported the theory of the reincarnation of the Pollock sisters. Even Mrs. Pollock, who was initially so adamantly against any suggestion of reincarnation, became convinced. Before her death in 1979, she admitted that she believed that her first two daughters were not really dead.

THE CASTE SYSTEM

Caste, the hereditary system of social classes found in India, is fundamental to the Hindu concept of reincarnation. After death, an individual is reborn into the life that he or she deserves — a good incarnation if virtuous, a bad one if wicked. Members of the higher castes are said to deserve all the privileges accorded them, while members of lower castes supposedly deserve the hardship and poverty of their lives.

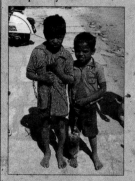

Beggar children

The god Brahma created the main castes. From his mouth came the highest caste, the Brahmans, which includes teachers and priests. From Brahma's arms came the Ksatriyas, the strong protectors, who are often in the army or police. From Brahma's thighs came the Vaisyas who work in business. From Brahma's feet came the Sudras, who serve the higher castes.

The untouchables

The Sudras and the untouchables are lowest on the social ladder and make up a third of the people of India. The castes are divided into thousands of sub-castes, such as goldsmiths, porters, carpenters, and sweepers. To this day, caste divisions affect Indian life. Efforts by the Indian government to outlaw the system have not succeeded.

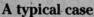

A Brahman
This 19th-century astronomer is of the highest caste.

REINCARNATION:
THE BIG DEBATE

Experts have unearthed some startling cases of children claiming to remember previous lives. Most of these occur in Eastern countries where reincarnation is part of the prevailing religion.

OVER A CENTURY'S RESEARCH into the possibility of life after death, and reincarnation in particular, has not allowed impartial investigators to come to any firm conclusions. However convincing some of the evidence may appear, it is still open to different interpretations.

One supporter of the case for reincarnation is Dr. Ian Stevenson, a Professor of Psychology at the University of Virginia Medical School. He and his fellow researchers have collected over 2,000 cases of alleged reincarnation experiences from around the world, especially from India, Sri Lanka, the Middle East, and Southeast Asia.

A typical case

Stevenson's extensive work has enabled him to outline a typical reincarnation profile. The subject is usually a child who, as soon as he is old enough to speak, says that he has other parents and a home in another village. He sometimes adds that he is married with children. When he is taken to the village, he gives a convincing display of having lived there before. For example, he finds the way to what he claims was his previous home from the outskirts of the village, comments correctly on changes made since his earlier life, and recognizes relatives hidden among crowds. Most incongruous but perhaps most compelling of all, he attempts to exert parental authority over the adults whom he claims to be his children. Memories of former lives usually fade when the child is around six.

In several cases, there is what appears to be physical evidence to support the theory of reincarnation. A rope mark, for example, appears on the neck of a child who claims to have met death by hanging in a previous life. In one case recorded by Stevenson, a child named Ravi Shankar claimed to be the reincarnation of a boy named Munna who had had his throat cut six

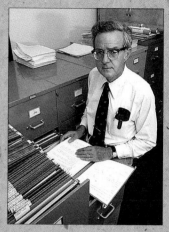

Dr. Ian Stevenson

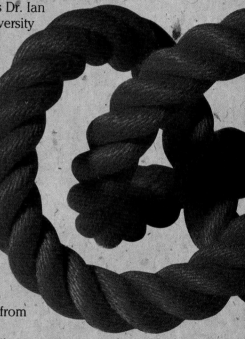

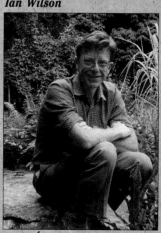

Ian Wilson

A rope mark appears on the neck of a child who claims to have met death by hanging in a previous life.

months before. Stevenson examined the boy and found an interesting birthmark on his neck: "Under the ridge of the chin...I observed a linear mark crossing the neck in a transverse direction....It looked much like an old scar of a healed knife wound."

The reincarnation question remains basically one that only personal faith or disbelief can answer. Among those who oppose the theory is the eminent British historian Ian Wilson, who has criticized Stevenson's findings on a number of fundamental points. Wilson points out that in compiling his research, Stevenson often had to rely on Buddhist and Hindu interpreters who were probably sincere, but not necessarily very objective. Second, Wilson highlights the lack of any uniformity in reincarnation claims. He says that it is significant that case histories from around the world seem to tie in with the different beliefs, religious and secular, of the various cultures. For example, Tlingit Alaskans believe that reincarnation can occur inside families while Asian Indians believe that it occurs only outside them. Intermissions between lives vary in time between 6 months and 19 years. Distances between present and former homes vary from half a mile to hundreds and even to thousands of miles. Wilson says it is also significant that

many former lives appear to have been in families wealthier and of a higher social class or caste than the reincarnate's present family.

Wilson argues convincingly from a study of cases in psychiatric literature that every element of the acting in past-life regressions can be explained in terms of the well-known psychological phenomenon of multiple personality. Subjects with this condition have different body images of themselves and produce different handwriting. Multiple personalities are thought to be caused by physical or mental traumas in early life, and the theory is that past-life regressions also have their basis in repressed traumas.

Many former lives appear to have been in families wealthier and of a higher social class than the present family.

For all the strength of his arguments, Wilson is forced to acknowledge that some cases of past-life regressions are undeniably impressive. The strange phenomenon is at present so little understood that a real basis in some kind of reincarnation cannot be ruled out as impossible.

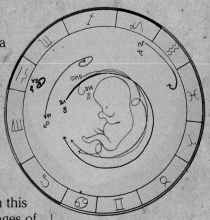

Heliocentric horoscope
This sun-centered astrological chart incorporates a person's past lives into the horoscope. Karma, or destiny, influences the individual's horoscope. Actions in a past life determine where, when, and to which parents he or she will be reborn.

Vendor from Varanasi
Street-sellers hold a low place in the Indian caste system.

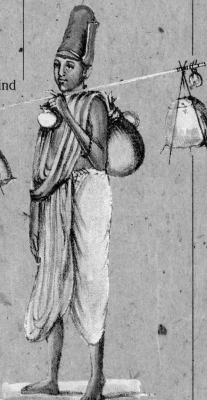

Shaping gold
Craftsmen such as this jeweler belonged to a sub-caste of the Sudra, the lowest Indian caste.

ALTERED IMAGES

Reincarnation is one way in which a body might be taken over by a spirit. But in fact it is only part of a much wider spectrum of experiences known as "possession."

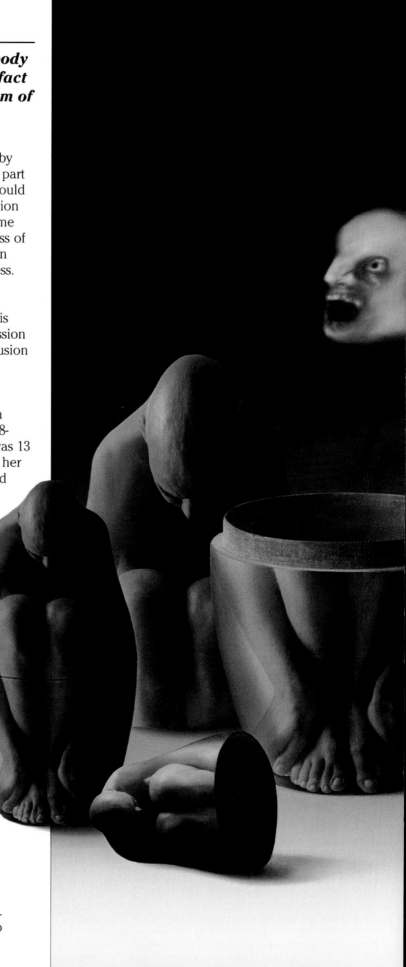

THE CONCEPT OF POSSESSION of human beings by either evil or good spirits is, or has been, a part of most religions. However, much of what would have been regarded in earlier centuries as infestation by demons is now attributed to mental illness. Some authorities maintain that all possession is a sickness of the mind. Other observers believe in a real division between spirit occupation and psychological illness.

Watseka Wonder case

Complete possession occurs only when someone is entirely occupied by an alien entity. Partial possession differs from this in that the person is aware of intrusion by a controlling outside character. One possible example of complete possession is the celebrated Watseka Wonder case of the 1870's. A girl named Lurancy Vennum was born in Watseka, Illinois, on April 16, 1864. Just over a year later, a neighbor, 18-year-old Mary Roff, died. In 1877, when Lurancy was 13 years old, she began hearing voices. She also told her family that she could see heaven, angels, and dead people whom she had known. Lurancy became possessed in turn by two distasteful personalities. One was an old hag, and the other was a dissolute young man.

Changing personalities

When Mary Roff's father heard of Lurancy's condition he became interested in the case. He suggested that she be put under the care of a medical hypnotist by the name of Dr. E. Winchester Stevens. Stevens claimed that he had managed to get through to the "sane and happy mind of Lurancy Vennum herself." This self said that an "angel" named Mary Roff wanted to come to her instead of the two unpleasant spirits. Lurancy remained herself and seemed to be aware of her body's occupation by intruders. However, a deeper possession followed in which her own personality disappeared entirely. A few days after speaking about Mary Roff, Lurancy became Mary so completely, in life and memory, that she went to live with the Roff family. The Mary Roff personality showed a knowledge of Mary's life and preferences well beyond what Lurancy could possibly have known. When she met friends or relatives of the Roffs who

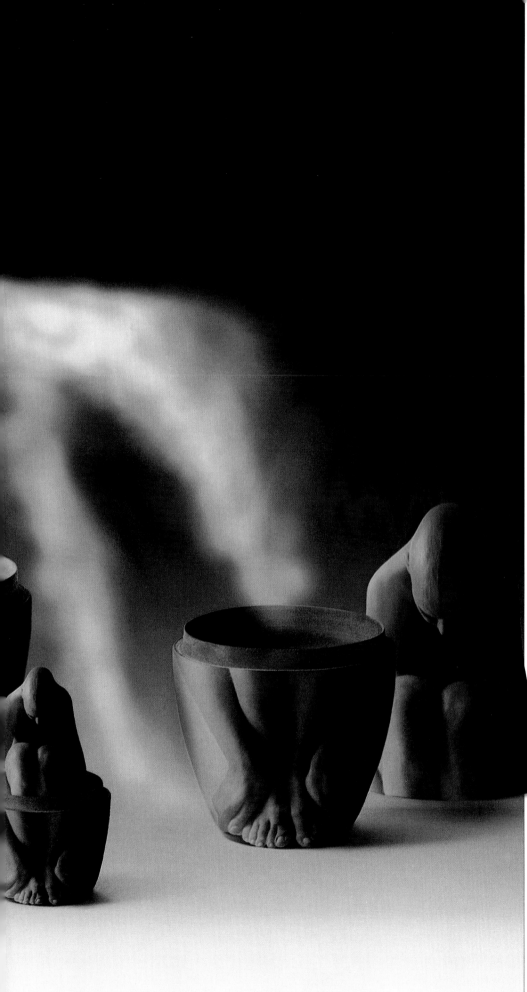

CONTORTED CHARACTERS

Three main characteristics are said to identify a case of possession. First and most obvious is facial distortion.

One victim in the 17th century was described as becoming: "completely unrecognizable, her glance furious, her tongue prodigiously large, long, and

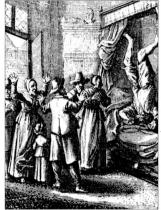

A 17th-century victim of demonic attack

hanging down out of her mouth." The second involves the voice. In one case an 11-year-old girl spoke in a deep, bass tone. The third is that the new voice speaks as if possessed by a completely different personality.

Compulsive movement

These phenomena are usually accompanied by unnatural movement — agitation of the limbs, with contortions. The victim seems to have no control over these compulsive actions. The body may bend backwards like a bow, and the victim is often impossible to restrain.

Animal intrusion

Possession may be by just one or several spirits. A common belief in some cultures is that the invading spirit is animal rather than human. In 1907 a Japanese case was reported in which a 17-year-old girl was recovering from a bad case of typhus. People in her room were discussing the fact that a fox had been seen near the house. "Hearing this, the girl felt a trembling in the body and was possessed. The fox had entered into her and spoke by her mouth."

had not been seen for years, she recognized them but remarked on how they had changed. The Lurancy personality was lost completely. She recognized none of her Vennum family nor her friends and was entirely ignorant of everything that Lurancy had known and done in her life. The Roff personality remained for about 100 days and then departed, to be replaced again by the Vennum character. During the time of possession, it would have been interesting to discover through hypnosis if a Vennum persona lurked deep below the Roff personality, but this was not tried with the girl.

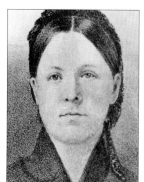

Lurancy Vennum

Lurancy's experience suggested that she was open to invasion by spirits. But there is no evidence that the old hag and young man ever existed. Perhaps the disembodied Mary Roff felt the need to inhabit a human body for a further short time. In this case, Mary Roff had to wait 12 years before a suitable trigger (her father's interest in Lurancy?) and recipient could be found. What is certain is that Lurancy never felt herself to be Mary reincarnated.

Mary Roff

Distant recollections
An individual who claims to have lived in previous incarnations does not believe that he or she is currently controlled by any former personalities. The person may, by "far memory," have some idea

Widespread belief
Tales of demonic possession were common in Christian countries during the Middle Ages. There are also examples from Jewish culture. Possession plays an important part in Indian Hindu legends and is a common belief in China and Japan as well.

of what it was like to be a peasant in ancient Egypt, a serving wench in Elizabethan England, a soldier in the Civil War, and a lady of fashion in the 1920's. While the person's present personality may be a product of all these

---

A woman regressed under hypnosis may remember loading and firing a cannon in the heat of battle during the Civil War.

---

diverse lives, it is different from any one of them. The person is a unique individual. He or she sees remembered past lives from the outside but also recalls them as his or her own. In this way a woman regressed under hypnosis may remember loading and firing a cannon in the heat of battle during the Civil War as something she had done herself, but still retains her own unique, contemporary personality.

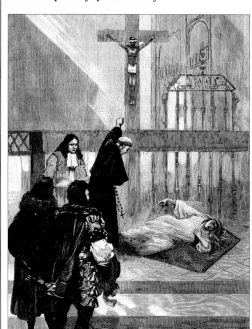

A contagious condition
The sight of other possessed people may prompt new cases of possession. A famous example occurred between 1632 and 1638 in the convent of the Little Ursulines in Loudun, France. This engraving shows one of the many exorcisms performed in order to free the possessed nuns. The epidemic spread outside the convent to affect people in Chinon, Nîmes, and Avignon. Cardinal Mazarin finally ended the outbreak by ordering that it should receive no more publicity.

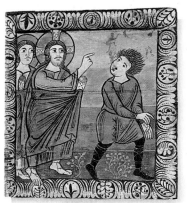

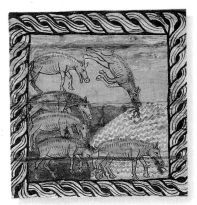

These 12th-century paintings depict Jesus driving devils into swine

VOLUNTARY POSSESSION

There are individuals, from Western mediums to Balinese trance dancers, who actually invite spirits to enter and possess their bodies.

MUCH POSSESSION involves unwilling victims, but there are also many cases of voluntary possession. In parts of Asia and Africa, there is a widespread belief in the ability of spirits to enter the human body. Shamans, or holy men, are believed to be able to influence these spirits. They can even invite demons to possess them in order to increase their healing powers.

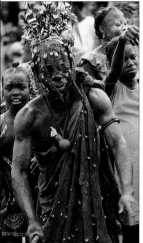

Nigerian shaman

In Sri Lanka, devil-dancing invites possession by demons to help cure disease. The following 19th-century account vividly recreates the scene — one that it is still possible to witness in Sri Lanka today: "Fantastically dressed, amidst the din of rattles, drums, and flutes, the conjurer of spirits begins his dance...as the music becomes quicker and louder, his excitement begins to rise....There is no mistaking that glare, those frantic leaps. He snorts, he stares, he gyrates. The demon has now taken bodily possession."

Good spirits

Possession may be by evil spirits, but there is possession by good spirits as well. The ancient Greeks took a wider view, regarding all inspiration, especially poetic, as a kind of possession. In some cultures today, it is believed that good spirits possess humans to help fight evil. An example of this is the trance dancing by graceful young girls in Bali.

Sensitive communicators

People described as sensitives (mediums) also accept possession voluntarily. They offer themselves as communicating channels between the spirit world and our own. At a séance, a sensitive settles into a waking state of total relaxation. This is probably a condition of very slight dissociation, something like light hypnosis. In this relaxed state, he or she may pass on

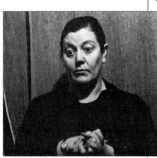

Eileen Garrett, a possessed medium

messages from the departed. If there is a "control," an entity who can communicate habitually through the medium, the sensitive may speak in a manner and personality different from his or her own. If in a trance, the medium may show the characteristics of the various communicating personalities as they take over in turn, speaking in different voices. Most people who claim to be possessed, either voluntarily or involuntarily, see themselves as different from the entities using their bodies. There is no sense that the other selves or communicating beings have existed as previous incarnations of the subjects.

Frenzied worship

A central part of voodoo worship is possession by the gods. Dance, chants, and drums all help to create an atmosphere in which a god and a human worshiper can become one. Worshipers enter a state of trance ending in complete collapse.

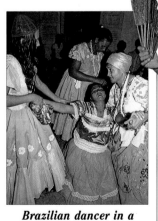

Brazilian dancer in a trance-induced swoon

Does possession by evil spirits cause disease? Many people around the world still believe it does. In some cultures there are special dances and ceremonies to chase away bad spirits. In Bali, it is believed that a divine spirit comes down to a village to help. The divine spirit reveals itself through a young person who dances with eyes closed in a trance. In the Sanghyang Dedari dance, two possessed young girls move gracefully through motions they cannot remember once out of the trance. They perform exactly the same movements even though their eyes are closed and they cannot watch each other as they dance.

Dance of angels

Sanghyang Dedari trance dancing ends when the girls fall to the ground in a swoon. A priest then prays beside them and blesses them with holy water. It is always young girls of about 10 or 11 who perform this dance, as virgins are thought most holy. *Sanghyang* is the name for the good spirit and *Dedari* means angel. The possessed girls who dance are much revered as special angels.

Balinese trance dancer

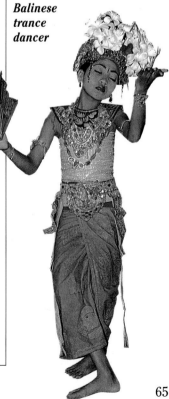

65

CHANGING IDENTITIES

In the case of alternating personalities, two people, each with a separate lifestyle and memory, take it in turns to inhabit a body. With multiple personalities, a number of different personalities are manifest in a body. If, for example, there are six such entities, the usual personality is unaware of the others. Personality number two knows of number one but not of the others, and so on. Only one personality is aware of all the others.

Taking turns

The different personalities take over the physical being at different times. They appear and disappear but do not succeed each other as they would in reincarnation.

Author and researcher Ian Wilson has suggested that Mrs. A. J. Stewart thinking she was James IV may be a classic case of multiple personality. Symptoms such as insomnia, black depressions, suicide attempts, and hysterical loss of speech are often found in the background of multiple-personality cases.

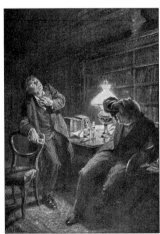

Dr. Jekyll and Mr. Hyde
Robert Louis Stevenson's book was first published in 1886. The good doctor changes into a dangerous and evil creature who alternates with his normal self. Someone who commits wicked deeds and yet may be loving to his or her family is typical of the alternating-personality idea.

An illustration of semi-possession is the experience of Mrs. A. J. Stewart, a novelist who wrote *Falcon: The Autobiography of His Grace, James IV, King of Scots*. Mrs. Stewart was convinced that she was the reincarnation of the Scottish king who, along with most of his noblemen, perished at the hands of the English in the battle of Flodden Field in 1513. Mrs. Stewart claimed she vividly remembered

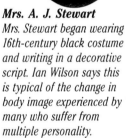

Mrs. A. J. Stewart
Mrs. Stewart began wearing 16th-century black costume and writing in a decorative script. Ian Wilson says this is typical of the change in body image experienced by many who suffer from multiple personality.

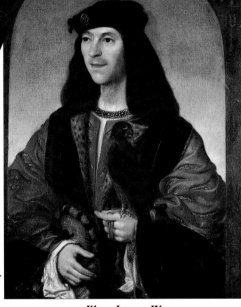

King James IV

her own death in the battle – but she never ceased to be herself. She remained conscious of being Mrs. Stewart who had been the Scottish king. She could therefore write about him in the first person without ceasing to be a 20th-century woman author.

There are several accounts of such "far memories" of adults in the literature of reincarnation. Joan Grant, born in 1907, wrote books describing more than 30 previous incarnations that she could remember – but she never ceased to be Joan Grant. Not everyone with such memories attributes them to reincarnation. A St. Louis author named

> ## She remained conscious of being Mrs. Stewart who had been the Scottish king.

Dorothy Wofford found herself writing lines of poetry that were later proved to be the work of the 17th-century New England poet Anne Broadbent. Investigation showed that Dorothy shared some unusual characteristics and tastes with Anne. It was suggested that unconscious mediumship or slight possession might provide alternative explanations to reincarnation in this case. Another explanation could be cryptomnesia, or hidden memory, through which some people remember every detail of a source, such as a book or a film, they thought they had only glanced at. This recall is often discovered under hypnosis.

Dr. Ian Stevenson, of the University of Virginia, studied numerous children who described past lives, many of which ended violently. One of his case histories involved a Belgian boy called Robert. When the boy saw a portrait of his Uncle Albert, who had died during the First World War, he was convinced that it was really of him. Robert was only three-and-a-half when a family friend filmed him using an old-style camera. As Robert ran past the camera he heard the loud "click-click-click" of the handle. "Don't," he screamed, "They killed me that way last time." He was unaware that his uncle had died in a hail of machine gun fire.

Stevenson suggests that spirits who die prematurely could be unwilling to give up life. The spirits may possess children whose unformed personalities allow them a temporary foothold. In time, these spirits may be pushed out as the child's personality grows stronger.

Casting out Evil

Rituals aimed at eradicating evil spirits are traditional in many cultures – and are still practiced all over the world.

XORCISM IS THE TRADITIONAL WAY of trying to rid someone of an unwelcome other being. An exorcist addresses the possessing spirit, ordering and persuading the demon to leave. Exorcisms are generally held at holy places but may take place at a victim's home.

The physical characteristics of the possessed may improve markedly after exorcism rituals. In 1865 two possessed young boys in Alsace suffered physical contortions. They entangled their legs and bent backwards with their bodies arched. Often they became bloated as if about to burst. Yellow foam, feathers, and seaweed were said to come out of their mouths. The demonic possession lasted four years before they were apparently freed by exorcism rites.

Sometimes rituals have no effect on the symptoms. One recent example involved Anneliese Michel, a young university student in Germany. In 1973 she showed signs of abnormal behavior, including violent rages and screaming. Although her symptoms were suggestive of mental illness, she did not consult a doctor. Her priest believed she was possessed by demons, and exorcism rituals began. Anneliese died in 1976 from malnutrition and dehydration. Her parents and

Nichiren in Japan
The belief that animal spirits can possess human beings is widespread in Japan. Exorcizing animal spirits is the special task of the Nichiren Buddhist sect. The possessed visit their temples in the hope of finding release.

two exorcists were charged with negligent homicide for not seeking conventional medical help.

The case of Anneliese is a reminder that some symptoms interpreted as possession may be linked to much more conventional medical conditions. For example, during a convulsive seizure, someone with epilepsy may become rigid, foam at the mouth, and show very rapid back-and-forth head movements.

Hysteria also shows symptoms that might be interpreted otherwise as possession. A hysterical person may entangle and disentangle his or her legs, and bend his or her body into a semicircle. This "hysterical arch" is frequently cited as a typical symptom of possession.

18-disease mask
This Sri Lankan mask shows a demon holding victims in his fists and mouth. The 18 fierce faces represent the demons responsible for disease. Possession by one of these demons will result in a particular sickness. To cure the sufferer, the appropriate demon must be exorcized during devil-dancing ceremonies.

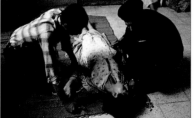

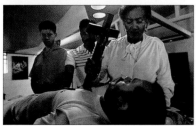

Modern rituals
Many modern Egyptians of all social classes believe in possession. They visit sanctuaries, like this one in Mit Damsis (above left), where exorcism is practiced regularly. Well-to-do Egyptians can afford to have exorcisms carried out at home. On the island of Réunion in the Indian Ocean, rituals are still performed by the local exorcist or tisanière *(left).*

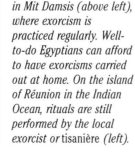

Devil-dancing

In the south of Sri Lanka, devil-dancing is the traditional way of casting out evil spirits. The ceremony for dealing with demons of disease is called *sanni yakuma*. It begins at dusk and ends at dawn the next day. The patient lies on a mat, overlooking the ritual.

At the start of the exorcism, demons are invited to appear. There are chants, beating of drums, and frantic masked dancing. The chief exorcist dresses as the chief of demons so that he can command other demons. Addressing each demon by name, the exorcist talks first in endearing terms, then implores, and finally threatens the demon. Eventually a demon may leave a sick person, after being bribed by offerings of food.

The eerie feeling of déjà vu is often strongly suggestive of reincarnation, but there are many other plausible explanations for it:

◆ Cryptomnesia: Our memories have a far greater capacity than we realize. Insignificant events from the past are recorded in the depths of our minds.

◆ Ego defense: Faced with threatening circumstances we may try to reassure ourselves that we have experienced them before. If we survived them the first time, surely we can do the same again.

◆ Redintegration: The sight of a familiar object in an unfamiliar scene could make us think the new location has been witnessed in the past.

◆ False memory: If our memories are not able to distinguish between two sets of similar circumstances or emotions, this could lead us to believe the new experience has happened before.

◆ Double functioning: We may experience a "double exposure" in the brain, whereby we see the same scene twice. Although only a split second elapses between the sightings, the brain extends the time so that it seems much longer.

◆ Diseases of the temporal lobe: Some diseases of the brain's temporal lobe cause disturbances of our sense of time.

◆ Paramnesia: As children we develop fantasies based on what we overhear from adults. When we become adults ourselves our real experiences often combine with dreams. If something we've imagined or dreamed actually happens, we may think it is from our previous experience.

A SENSE OF DÉJÀ VU

Déjà vu is the name for what is probably the most common psychic experience of all — the feeling that "I have seen or experienced this before."

THE TERM "DÉJÀ VU" was first used by F. L. Arnaud in 1896. But references to the sensation of repeating an experience can be found as early as the Roman poet Ovid (43 B.C. – A.D. 18). Charles Dickens described the phenomenon in his novel *David Copperfield*: "We have all some experience of a feeling that comes over us occasionally of what we are saying and doing having been said and done before...of our knowing perfectly what will be said next, as if we suddenly remembered it."

Charles Dickens

Vivid memories

A striking example of déjà vu was recorded in 1970 by Martin Ebon in his book *Reincarnation in the Twentieth Century*. In 1966, a 26-year-old German woman named Inge Ammann was on a touring vacation with her husband. As they were driving through countryside near Germany's border with Czechoslovakia, Inge suddenly felt that the area was very familiar. On turning into a side road that led through woodland to a village, she exclaimed "I've lived here before. I know exactly where everything is."

Inge felt sure that before the Second World War she had been a peasant girl living with her parents and two brothers on a farm in that very place. When Inge and her husband arrived in the village, she was able to guide him around its streets. She seemed to know

She seemed to know every old building in the hamlet and identified the house where she believed she had been born as a peasant girl.

every old building in the hamlet and identified the house where she believed she had been born as a peasant girl. She also recognized the old innkeeper. He confirmed her story and remembered that a family like the one she described had owned a local farm, which was now run by the surviving brother. The parents and other brother were dead. The innkeeper also recalled the tragic death of the family's young daughter. She had been kicked to death by a horse in a stable. As the innkeeper told the story, Inge experienced instant, vivid recall of the awful event, and cried out in anguish at the painful memory of it.

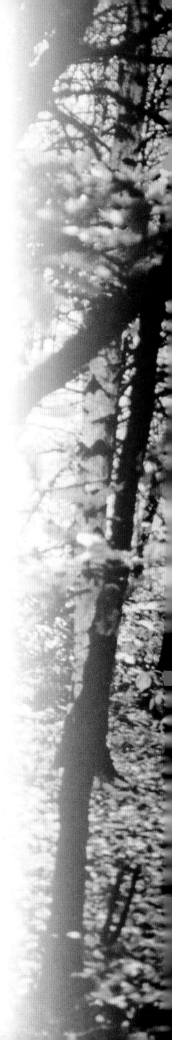

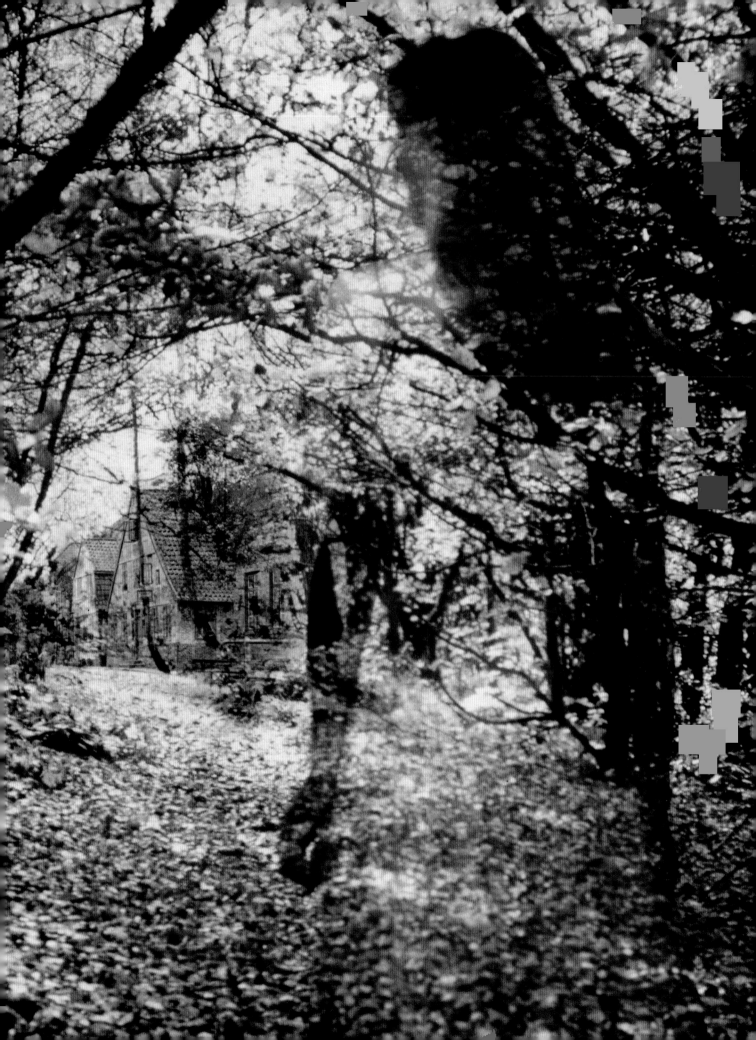

CHARTING PAST LIVES

Some astrologers believe that astrology may provide the key to past lives. Locked within each birth chart are pointers to the historical periods in which we have lived.

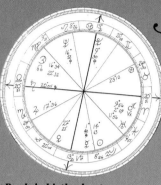

Paulo's birth chart

Emilia Lorenz committed suicide but returned at a séance to tell her mother that she wanted to come back, this time as a boy. Senhora Lorenz later gave birth to a son, Paulo. He insisted on wearing girl's clothing and showed other signs of being Emilia reincarnated. But he was never happy, and he too killed himself. Similarities between Emilia and Paulo abound — but were they one soul?

Thornton cast birth and death charts for them both. She looked for indications that they had shared one soul. Thornton tested various theories of the link between past lives and astrology against her readings. None of them worked exactly, but there were far more parallels between the charts than one would expect.

*S*INCE ANCIENT TIMES, various mystics have held the view that man is ruled by the stars and the planets and that the cosmos is reflected within him. Astrologers and psychics have long believed that this cosmic connection means that astrology can be used to reveal past lives. Many reputable astrologers, however, believe that this connection between astrology and past lives will never be proved. Others, equally eminent, think that they already have the answer.

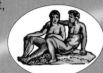

Gemini (6580 B.C. – 5500 B.C.)
The ancient Mediterranean.

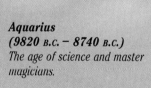

Cancer (8740 B.C. – 7660 B.C.)
The destruction of Atlantis.

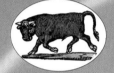

Taurus (4420 B.C. – 3340 B.C.)
The rise and fall of ancient empires.

Aries (2260 B.C. – 1180 B.C.)
The Old Testament.

Pisces (100 B.C. – A.D. 980)
The Christian age.

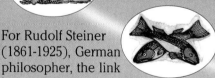

Aquarius (9820 B.C. – 8740 B.C.)
The age of science and master magicians.

For Rudolf Steiner (1861-1925), German philosopher, the link between a previous life and the current life was simple — a "remarkable correlation" exists between the present life's birth chart and a past life's death chart. Steiner also thought that after death the soul journeyed around the planets adding to its spiritual development, prior to its reincarnation on earth. He believed that the birth chart told the story of these travels. Edgar Cayce, thought by some to be the greatest psychic of the 20th century, also believed that astrology held the key to past lives. Like Steiner, Cayce believed the soul embarked on a planetary journey after death, influencing the next life.

A journey through time
It is the opinion of many astrologers that time is a spiral. Each reincarnation is a moment in time; each horoscope reveals the soul's destiny in the future and its links with the past. Knowing which sign Saturn is in in your birth chart may reveal which astrological age was important to you in the past. To support this theory, astrologer Marc Robertson has assigned the labels used here to astrological ages.

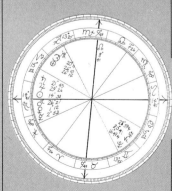

Emilia's birth chart

"Our astrological influences from the planets, or dimensions we have inhabited, will be good or bad, weak or strong, according to experiences we have had here, and how we handled problems," wrote Cayce.

Some astrologers, among them Marc Robertson and Tad Mann, have gone further, attempting to actually decode the birth chart. Robertson believes that the key lies in the place of the planet Saturn in the chart. For instance, where Saturn is in Leo, Robertson says the individual had an important life during the age of Atlantis (10,900 B.C. – 9820 B.C.); or where Saturn is in Pisces, a life governed by the Christian age (100 B.C. – A.D. 980) could be expected.

Other astrologers are skeptical of a simple solution to such a complex problem. For them, astrology must work with other skills — psychic powers or hypnotic regression — to uncover past lives.

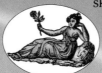

Leo
(10,900 B.C. – 9820 B.C.)
The golden age of Atlantis.

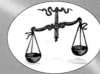

Virgo
(A.D. 980 – A.D. 2060)
The age of scholasticism.

Libra (1180 B.C. – 100 B.C.)
Classical Greece and Rome.

Scorpio (3340 B.C. – 2260 B.C.)
Ancient Egypt and the East.

Sagittarius (5500 B.C. – 4420 B.C.)
The age of wandering tribes.

Capricorn (7660 B.C. – 6580 B.C.)
The post-Atlantean world.

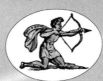

With a hypnotist, English astrologer Penny Thornton regressed people to four past lives and cast charts for each of the lives, including the present one. She claimed that the readings showed significant correlations between the various past lives and helped the subjects deal with problems in their present lives.

Learning about past lives is more than a complex puzzle or a parlor game. Devotees claim that knowing about one's past lives may reveal a great deal about how to solve problems in the present. Birth charts contain messages that no one can afford to ignore.

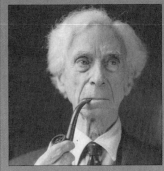

Bertrand Russell

LINKED LIVES
Astrologer Robert Powell looks to Saturn to find the key to our past lives. By charting the relationship between the positions of Saturn and the Sun in the birth chart, Powell has located past lives for a number of famous people.

For example, according to Powell, 20th-century philosopher Bertrand Russell's chart reveals that in the past he has been

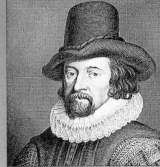

Francis Bacon

incarnated as Sir Francis Bacon (1561-1626), the English politician, and Harun al-Rashid (A.D. 763 – A.D. 809), a caliph or ruler of Baghdad. The three men could not be more different — yet they are all linked by Saturn.

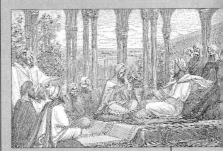

Harun al-Rashid

71

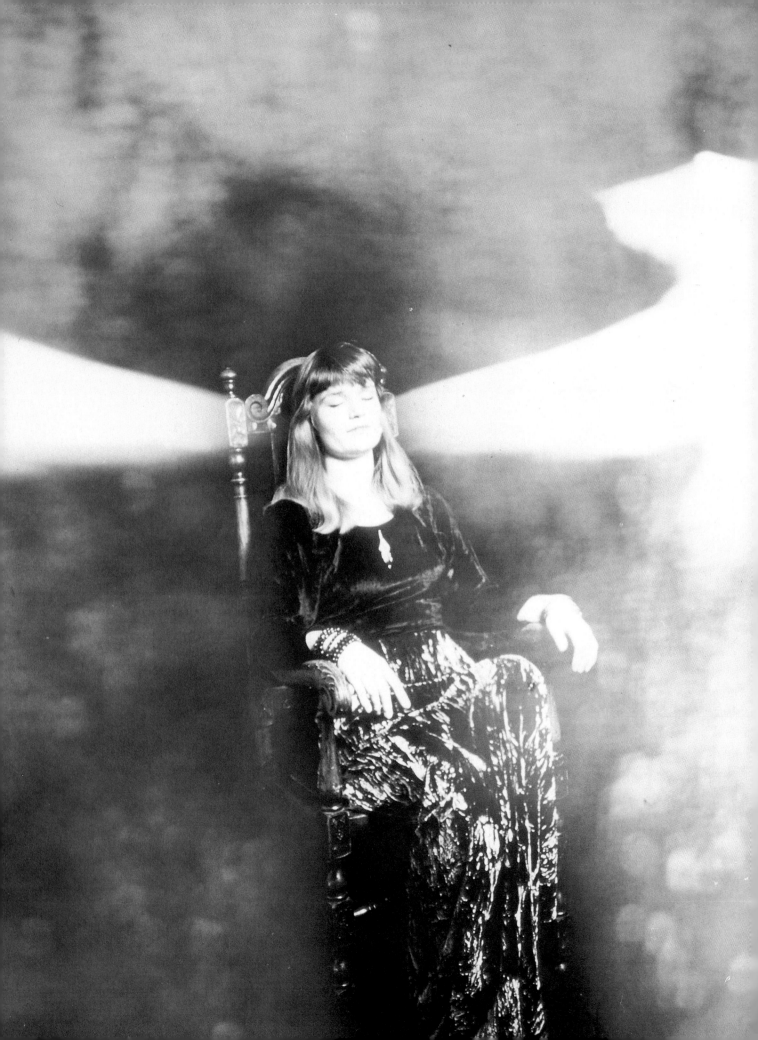

CHAPTER THREE

DO THE DEAD SPEAK?

Following the birth of the spiritualist movement in the mid-1800's, psychical researchers began ingenious tests of the paranormal. Many spiritualists believed that these investigations would prove the reality of life after death. But absolute proof is still elusive.

In 1848, inexplicable rapping noises were heard in the home of the Fox family in Hydesville, New York. The two young Fox sisters, Catherine and Margaretta, started to "communicate" with the mysterious rappings. The girls claimed that they were conversing with spirits from the next world. News of the phenomenon spread quickly and within two years the sisters had become national celebrities. The Fox girls and their claim of

HIDDEN GUIDANCE

A ouija board is a flat board on which the letters of the alphabet, the numbers one through nine, and the words "yes" and "no" are printed. It was invented in Baltimore in 1891 by Elijah J. Bond. The board is designed to provide a way of contacting those who have departed this world for "the other side."

Participants sit around the board and formulate questions, while lightly touching an upturned glass or a pointer mounted on castors. All who take part physically touch each other or the pointer so that it is a group effort. The pointer then spells out responses, moving as if directed by a strange invisible force.

In 1966 Parker Brothers Inc. bought all rights to the ouija board, and since then millions have been sold.

Planchette boards

A planchette board is slightly different from a ouija board. It consists of a movable, triangular-shaped platform which is supported on two sides by castors. The third side holds a pencil that makes contact with paper on the surface underneath. As with the ouija board, one or more people lightly touch the planchette. This appears to move about of its own volition, writing out spirit messages.

Using a ouija board, 1903

contact with the dead marked the start of the spiritualist movement.

However, their feats were soon overshadowed by far more impressive examples of contact between this world and the next. Tables began to levitate. Strange lights glowed. Objects were produced from thin air and dropped into sitters' laps. Invisible hands caressed investigators, played musical instruments, and even wrote messages on sealed slates. Voices were heard, sometimes several speaking simultaneously and occasionally in foreign tongues. And then came the ultimate proof in the eyes of many — the materialization of ectoplasm and the emergence of a visitor from the next world.

According to spiritualists, ectoplasm is the mysterious substance that appears in an abstract, chiffonlike form before taking on the shape of a spirit visitor.

All these phenomena had two things in common. They invariably took place in darkened séance rooms, and they required the presence of a medium.

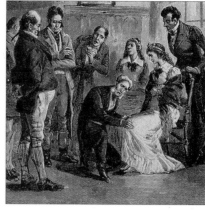

Humble beginnings
In 1851 some skeptical researchers announced that the Fox sisters were "popping" their knee joints and claiming the sounds as spirit communications. In 1888 Margaretta Fox revealed that their mediumship had been a complete fraud — but she withdrew the confession a year later.

Not surprisingly, there were many critics who dismissed these mediums as charlatans. A number of conjurers earned a good living by using trickery to produce "spirit phenomena" on stage.

Prominent believers

Although some mediums were known to be fraudulent, many prominent people in the United States and Europe became convinced that mediums had enabled them to communicate with departed friends and relatives. Queen Victoria is reputed to have held séances at Osborne House on the Isle of Wight. Some spiritualists maintain that her Scottish manservant, John Brown, was a medium through whom she regularly received messages from her dead husband, Prince Albert. European royalty and the Russian czars were also fascinated by the phenomena of spiritualism. The services of Daniel Dunglas Home, who was one of the most famous of 19th-century mediums, were much in demand throughout Europe.

Mind games
This is a modern ouija board, but the concept has ancient roots. As long as 4,000 years ago, the Chinese used a branched bough to communicate with spirits. When held by two people in the presence of spirits, the bough would move independently, spelling out spirit messages in the sand.

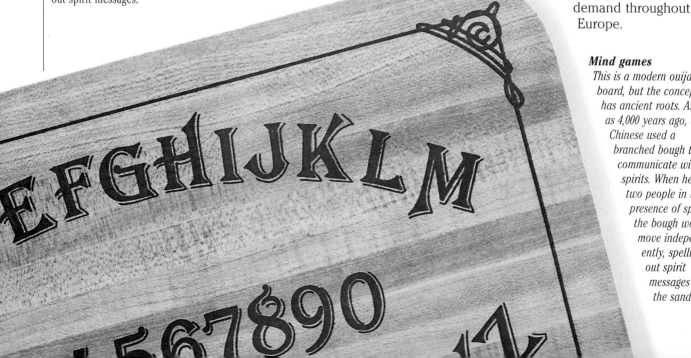

EFGHIJKLM

567890

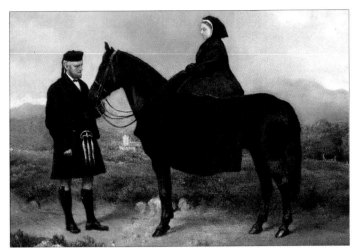

Queen Victoria and her servant John Brown

In the mid-1980's, a University of Chicago National Opinion Research Council survey concluded that almost half of American adults believed they had been in contact with someone who had died.

Unknown forces
Scottish-American Daniel Dunglas Home was a well-known medium who came under thorough scientific investigation. The Victorian scientist William Crookes concluded that Home did possess some powerful psychic force.

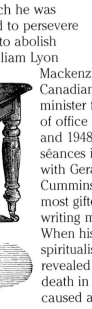

Home and others of his time are now referred to as "physical" mediums. The phenomena they seem to have produced were actual manifestations. There are very few physical mediums today. Skeptics point out that physical mediums may have gone out of style because their claims could not withstand rigorous scientific tests by modern recording equipment. Spiritualism now involves much more activity by "mental" mediums, whose claims are harder to authenticate. Powers such as clairvoyance, clairaudience, trance, and automatic writing allow these mediums to see and hear spirits and to convey information to their sitters. At its best, mental mediumship can be extremely convincing. For example, when a medium is in a trance, the contacting spirit may speak in a voice like that of a person now dead.

Political interest
In addition to royalty, prominent political figures have been interested in spirit communications. Abraham Lincoln attended several séances, during which he was encouraged to persevere in his fight to abolish slavery. William Lyon Mackenzie King, Canadian prime minister for three terms of office between 1921 and 1948, attended séances in London with Geraldine Cummins, one of the most gifted automatic writing mediums. When his interest in spiritualism was revealed after his death in 1950, it caused a sensation.

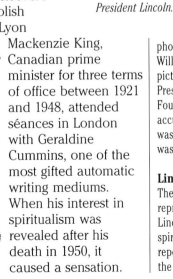

Spiritual counsel
Medium Nettie Colburn advising President Lincoln.

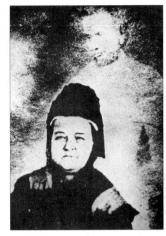

Deathly pose
Mary Todd Lincoln with her husband in a photo taken after his assassination.

SPIRITUAL REASSURANCE
Abraham Lincoln attended a number of séances following the death of his son, Willie, several of which were conducted by teenage medium Nettie Colburn. She stated that at one of these séances, held in December 1862, the spirits made a strong plea for Lincoln to proceed with the abolition of slavery.

Psychic photo
In 1865, soon after Lincoln was assassinated, his widow, Mary Todd Lincoln, visited a Boston psychic photographer by the name of William Mumler. She took away a picture of herself with the President standing behind her. Four years later Mumler was accused of being a swindler and was brought to trial, but the case was dismissed.

Lincoln's ghost
The ghostly photograph does not represent the end of Abraham Lincoln's involvement with the spirit world. His specter is reported to walk the corridors of the White House to this day.

ECTOPLASM

Ectoplasm is the outer layer surrounding the protoplasm of a cell. In the world of spiritualism, it is also the fleshy substance that appears as spirits take material form. When spiritualism was at its peak, flows of ectoplasm were all the rage.

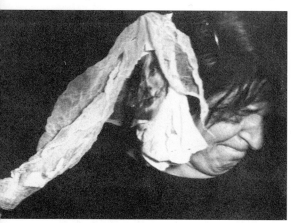

Materializing spirits
A medium exudes ectoplasm from her ear. A small face is visible, the start of a full materialization.

The material seemed to emerge from a medium's body, usually from the mouth and nose. One Canadian medium called Mary M. was known for producing ectoplasm in which human faces appeared. It was taboo to touch ectoplasm, but those who dared said it felt like chiffon cloth.

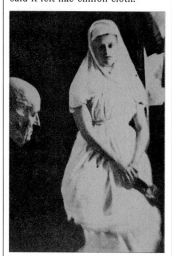

Spirit double
Medium Florence Cook materialized the spirit "Katie," seen here in ectoplasmic robes.

With the passage of time, new forms of spirit phenomena emerged. For example, spirit photography and psychic art offered the bereaved an opportunity to receive portraits of their loved ones. In the early 1900's the Chicago-based sisters Lizzie and May Bangs claimed to be able to "materialize" pictures onto canvas without the need to paint. Their results have been likened to airbrush techniques, which were developed much later. In some cases the picture was produced before the sitters' eyes in as little as eight minutes. Most psychic artists simply paint portraits of the dead they claim to see clairvoyantly.

Scientific study

Concerned that all of these psychic phenomena were open to abuse and trickery, some investigators turned either to spontaneous events or to the laboratory in their search for conclusive proof of life after death. Apparitions of the dead, and the living, were among the first subjects examined by the Society for Psychical Research, formed in Britain in 1882. Later researchers decided to study deathbed visions and out-of-body experiences in attempts to establish the truth about man's nature and the possibility that part of us, a soul, survives death. Sir William Crookes, Sir Oliver Lodge, and Sir William Barrett were among the many scientists who became convinced of the existence of a life after death as a result of their studies.

Popular support

In the century and a half that has elapsed since the emergence of spiritualism, hundreds of thousands of people have been convinced that they too have been in touch with spirits in

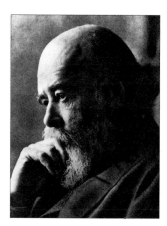

Life goes on
Sir Oliver Lodge was a tireless researcher into the unknown, and he became president of the Society for Psychical Research in 1932. As a result of his extensive investigations, Lodge felt certain that life continues after death.

> Since the emergence of spiritualism, hundreds of thousands of people have been convinced that they too have been in touch with spirits in the next world.

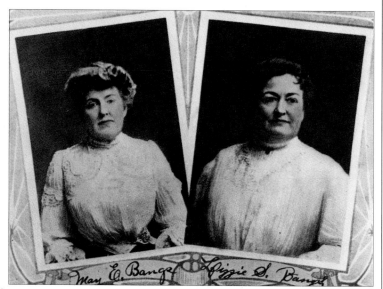

The Bangs sisters
In 1905 a man went to the Bangs sisters and asked them to materialize a portrait of his dead father — and they did. The sisters had never seen or heard of the father, but simply asked the man to concentrate deeply on his father's features, seeing them in his mind. First a faint shadow appeared on canvas, and then the likeness became clearer. The sisters apparently used no brushes or paints in producing these extraordinary pictures.

the next world. However, critical sense may have been clouded by grief or by the very understandable desire to believe that one's own death does not bring oblivion. The countless cases of known fraud add a further note of caution to the issue.

Communication — or ESP?

It could be that mental mediums are simply displaying skills in extrasensory perception (ESP). In the 20th century, scientists such as Dr. J. B. Rhine, working at Duke University, North

---

Researchers have studied deathbed visions and out-of-body experiences to establish the truth about man's nature and the possibility that part of us, a soul, survives death.

Carolina, have focused their research on telepathy and ESP. Although their results have impressed other parapsychologists, science in general is skeptical of their findings. This is due to the inability of many psychical researchers to produce an experiment that can guarantee results or be replicated to order. If we rule out fraud and self-deception, we must still decide whether a spirit communication is what it purports to be. Or do mediums use ESP to gather information from the minds of sitters, dressing everything up as messages from the grave?

A helping hand

This fake hand was used by equally fake spiritualists, who claimed that it was part of a materialized spirit.

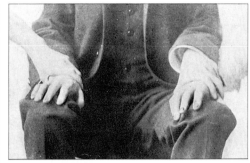

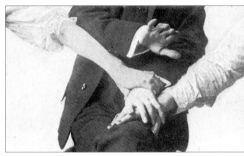

Trusting hands

Using a combination of sleight-of-hand and dexterity, it is relatively easy for a medium to fool his fellow sitters. Here, those sitting on either side of the medium in a suitably darkened room remain convinced that they are each holding a different hand. But the medium, having removed his right hand on some pretext, quickly crosses his legs and regrasps his neighbor's hand with his left hand, leaving his right hand free to go about its trickery.

Exposure time

M. Lamar Keene has confessed to having worked as a fake medium. Here he demonstrates his fraudulent practices by producing a dramatic excess of phony "ectoplasm." It seems likely that in the expectant atmosphere of a séance room, witnesses were prepared to believe anything. Keene reports that after a good weekend he would come away "with a suitcase full of money."

FACTORY OF DREAMS

In his book *The Belief in a Life After Death*, C. J. Ducasse, a philosopher at Brown University, Providence, Rhode Island, reported finding what must be "one of the most remarkable factories in the world."

"Here is everything a medium needs to perform a spiritualist séance, and false mediums from all over the world place orders through this firm. These false mediums, who operate in most countries, then appear to make contact with the 'other side,' and let ingenuous, faithful, mourning people believe that they are meeting dead relatives, while in fact the manifestations were bought by postal order from a firm in the U.S.A....

"We sent for material for an hour-long trick séance and can assure you that the effects are quite fantastic."

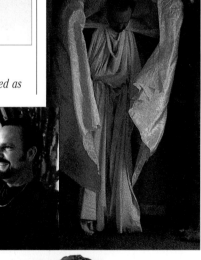

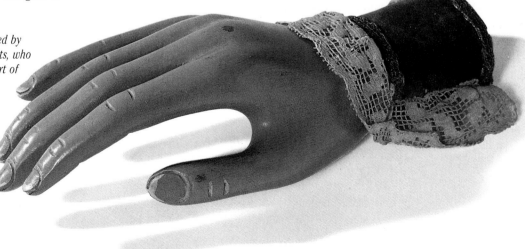

Helen Duncan was a very popular psychic in the 1930's and 1940's. She traveled around Britain holding séances in homes and spiritualist churches. Thousands of people were convinced that the dead could come back in a physical form. There was much controversy over whether the ectoplasm she materialized was genuine or some kind of fraud.

Brought to trial

In 1943 Mrs. Duncan was prosecuted under the Witchcraft Act of 1735, found guilty, and sentenced to nine months' imprisonment for "dishonesty."

Mrs. Duncan's trial prompted a change in the law, and in 1951 the Witchcraft Act was replaced by the Fraudulent Mediums Act. However, in 1956 police again raided a séance conducted by Mrs. Duncan.

Spiritualists regard it as dangerous to interrupt a séance, and in this particular case Mrs. Duncan suffered terrible pain. She died five weeks later.

Restricted information

Alan Crossley, a psychic investigator, has said that Mrs. Duncan was prosecuted because she was a security risk. "During the Second World War servicemen killed in action were regularly manifesting at her séances. Relatives of these men were startled when their sons told them that they were killed at such and such a place...or sailors named the ship on which they had died....The Admiralty didn't release such information for as long as three months. They were alarmed that through Mrs. Duncan's mediumship, the men were manifesting and telling the world about it within hours of the tragedy. They had to stop her."

SPIRITUAL CONTACT

Are there any cases of spirit communication that offer enough hard evidence to satisfy the sternest critics? Or are all otherworldly messages as unreliable as the skeptics claim?

THE PIONEERS OF PSYCHICAL RESEARCH were well aware that providing proof of life after death was beset with problems. It seemed that no matter how strong the evidence, there was always someone who could come up with some alternative explanation, such as telepathy or fraud.

Frederic W. H. Myers, a brilliant scholar, author of *Human Personality and Its Survival of Bodily Death*, and one of the founders of the Society for Psychical Research (SPR) came up with an answer...from the next world. Soon after his death in Rome in January 1901, mediums began to receive communications that seemed to come from the dead man.

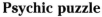

Helen Duncan

Psychic puzzle

Myers may have decided that the best way to prove that he still existed was to send a series of messages through different mediums. These messages were meaningless on their own, but impressive when put together. He never suggested such a project before his death, but it became a real possibility when the SPR's research officer, Miss Alice Johnson, began to detect unexpected, intricate, and complementary information in automatic writing scripts sent to her by mediums from around the world. The fragments often contained references to ancient Greek or Latin quotations.

The psychics who participated in these cross-correspondences were respectable individuals. Most were non-professional mediums who worked under pseudonyms. They included Rudyard Kipling's sister, Mrs. Alice Fleming in India; Mrs. Winifred Coombe-Tennant, a delegate to the League of Nations, in London; Mrs. Margaret Verrall, a lecturer in classics at Newnham College, Cambridge, England; Mrs. Verrall's daughter Helen; and Mrs. Leonora Piper, a trance medium from Boston, Massachusetts.

Myers seems to have explained the purpose of this psychic puzzle in a message received by Mrs. Verrall: "Record the bits and when fitted they will make the whole...I will give the words between you neither alone can read but together they will give the clue he wants."

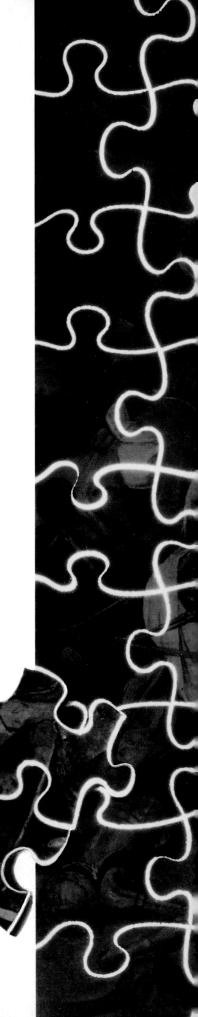

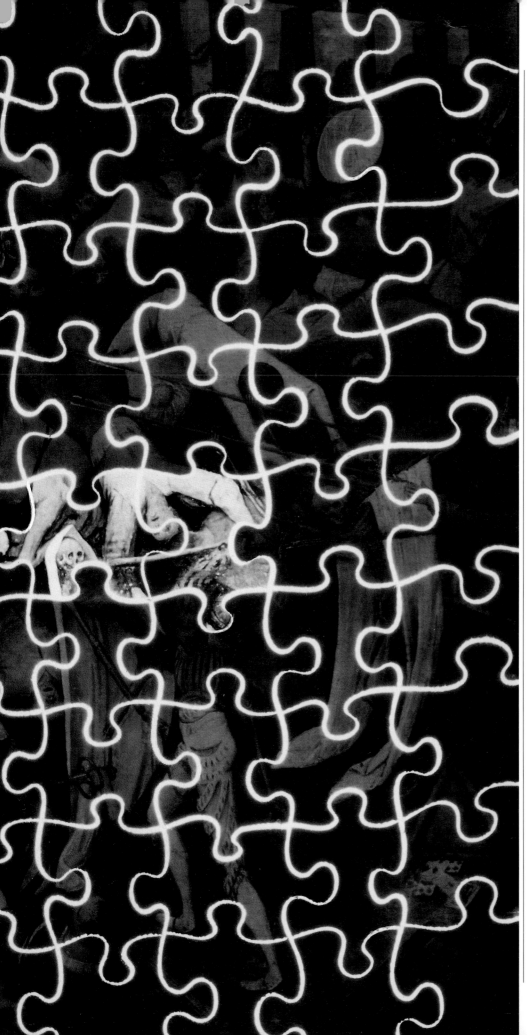

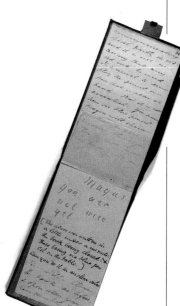

Taking notes
*An example of automatic
writing from the 1870's.*

AUTOMATIC WRITING

Automatic writing is handwriting,
or typewriting, made without the
writer's conscious control.
Mediums who perform automatic
writing claim to receive dictation
from spirit beings.

Cross-correspondences

Sometimes the automatic message
comes in fragments to a number
of different mediums. Each
fragment seems meaningless on
its own, unless combined with
others to make up a whole
message. In some cases the
messages contain obscure
references, the point of which is
revealed by a key word or clue.

Change of style

In many instances automatic
writing fragments appear in
handwriting that differs markedly
from the usual script of the
medium. This seems consistent
with the fact that mediums adopt
a different tone of voice when
receiving spoken messages from
the beyond.

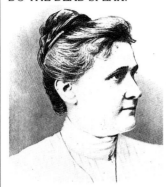

Medium Leonora Piper

POSITIVE PROOF
William James was an American psychologist and philosopher who pioneered much psychical research. In 1885 he became impressed by medium Leonora Piper of Boston and studied her over the next 12 years. He concluded that she was quite genuine. "I am persuaded of the medium's honesty and the genuineness of her trance. I now believe her to be in the possession of a power as yet unexplained."

During one séance, Piper told James that his aunt in New York had died that morning at 12:30. When he returned home, James found a telegram informing him that his Aunt Kate had passed away a few minutes after midnight.

Non-believer converted
Dr. Richard Hodgson worked with James and later wrote that he joined the investigation of Mrs. Piper with the idea of disproving her. "I entered the house...not believing in the continuance of life after death, and today I simply say, I believe."

Childhood experience
Mediums often suffered traumatic childhoods. Leonora's young life was unremarkable until the age of eight. She then felt a blow on her right ear and heard a hissing sound, followed by a voice which said: "Aunt Sara not dead but with you still." The event coincided with the actual death of the aunt.

Leonora Piper was one of several mediums said to receive scripts from Frederic Myers.

This communication gave the mediums the idea that the various messages they had received would only make sense when pieced together. Among the mediums only Mrs. Verrall and her daughter had the knowledge of classical languages needed to understand the detailed references contained in the messages. A team of highly qualified researchers at the SPR took over the work of deciphering the communications.

Ave Roma Immortalis was one of the least complicated of the correspondences. On the 2nd, 4th, and 5th of March, 1906, Mrs. Verrall received three scripts that purported to be from Myers. The first contained a line of Latin verse taken from the second book of the *Aeneid*, describing the fall of Troy. Apart from a reference to "the Stoic persecutor," which she took to be a reference to the Roman emperor Marcus Aurelius, Mrs. Verrall was unable to make sense of the remainder of the material. She was merely informed by the communicator that she would soon receive a message from another woman.

Hail immortal Rome
The next message came through on March 7. Mrs. Holland, who was totally unaware of the existence of Mrs. Verrall's scripts, received the following from Myers: "*Ave Roma Immortalis.* How could I make it any clearer without giving her the clue?" When the combined scripts were examined by an expert, it was discovered that they outlined a brief history of Rome, one of Myers's favorite subjects.

As well as assembling these post-mortem jigsaws, the researchers — notably J. G. Piddington in London and George B. Dorr in the United States —

> # The Myers scripts have been the subject of intense and continuing research.

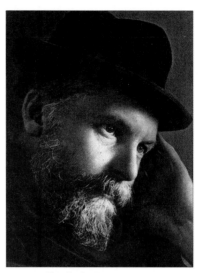

Frederic W. H. Myers
His scripts suggest that communication with the dead is a real possibility.

began putting classical questions to Myers via the mediums. The replies, often in the form of anagrams, were as impressive as the unsolicited messages. Frank Podmore, one of the most skeptical investigators, considered the case to be "perhaps the strongest evidence yet obtained identifying any communicator."

Persuasive scripts
The Myers cross-correspondence scripts were produced for almost 30 years and have been the subject of intense and continuing research. Communications also came from some of Myers's research colleagues who died a few years after him. There is obviously no certainty in claims of this kind, but the evidence that messages did indeed come from Myers after his death is striking and persuasive.

Over three years after Myers's death, Piddington deposited an envelope with the SPR, intending to attempt to communicate its contents after his own death. Soon afterwards six mediums relayed messages referring to this supposedly secret experiment that they claimed came from Myers.

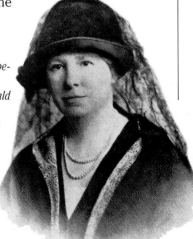

Discreet
Winifred Coombe-Tennant was medium to Gerald W. Balfour. She worked under a pseudonym — her true identity remaining a secret until after her death.

Daylight impressions

In addition to her involvement in the Myers cross-correspondence case, Mrs. Coombe-Tennant produced a long series of equally remarkable automatic scripts between 1912 and 1930. These were made up of what she called her "daylight impressions." As words formed in her mind she would write them down. She was convinced that the messages which began to unfold came from the

> "These automatic scripts are a very important addition to the vast mass of such material which suggests that certain human beings have survived the death of their physical bodies."
>
> **Prof. C. D. Broad**

spirit world. The messages repeatedly spelled out the request that someone called Gerald W. Balfour should attend one of Mrs. Coombe-Tennant's sittings. Gerald Balfour had been SPR president in 1906 and 1907, and was the younger brother of Arthur, the first earl of Balfour, an eminent politician who served as British prime minister, first lord of the admiralty, and foreign secretary.

Mrs. Coombe-Tennant initially resisted the request to have Gerald Balfour present at a sitting, but eventually agreed. During the séances that followed it became apparent that the spirit of a woman was trying to contact Gerald's brother, Arthur. Several other mediums involved in the cross-correspondence case had received similar messages. In 1916, in response to repeated pleas in Mrs. Coombe-Tennant's scripts, Gerald persuaded his brother to attend one of her séances.

In 1935 Gerald published a paper in the SPR's *Proceedings* about the sittings with Mrs. Coombe-Tennant. He explained that he could not disclose everything that had happened because some of it was too personal. The material finally came to light in 1960

when the countess of Balfour, Arthur's niece, contributed her own paper to the SPR's *Proceedings*. This text entitled "The Palm Sunday Case" detailed Arthur Balfour's love for a young woman who died of typhus on March 21, 1875. The countess believed that this was the woman who so desperately sought to communicate with Gerald and Arthur.

The death of Mrs. Coombe-Tennant in 1956 does not appear to have put an end to her interest in communications through mediums. Miss Geraldine Cummins, a well known automatic writer and medium, claimed to have received a series of 40 scripts from Mrs. Coombe-Tennant between August 1957 and March 1960.

The full story behind the scripts was published in Cummins's book *Swan on a Black Sea*. The scripts began when the SPR's honorary secretary, Mr. W. H. Salter, asked Miss Cummins to take part in an experiment. When she agreed, he simply sent her the name of Major Henry Tennant, who hoped to receive a message from his mother. The resulting scripts tell of Mrs. Coombe-Tennant's life, relationships with others, her psychic work, and include names, dates, and other details.

Arthur James Balfour

Doubting critics

In his analytical foreword to Cummins's book, Prof. C. D. Broad, Fellow of Trinity College, Cambridge, England, expressed the belief that "these automatic scripts are a very important addition to the vast mass of such material which *prima facie* suggests rather strongly that certain human beings have survived the death of their physical bodies."

Despite these and other impressive communications, critics have continued to be dismissive. Francis Clive-Ross, editor of an occult magazine called *Tomorrow*, wrote in 1963 that one of the strongest arguments against spiritualism was that its messages were of little value.

A POLITICIAN'S LOVE

The Palm Sunday story is a romantic tale linking Arthur James Balfour (later to become British prime minister) to a girl named Mary Catherine Lyttelton, who died of typhus on Palm Sunday in 1875 at the age of 24. Balfour was desolate at her death and, two years later, he had a silver box made to hold a lock of her hair.

Message of love

In the early 1900's a group of mediums received various messages from the other side, all of which appeared to be from Mary Lyttelton. She was trying to contact Arthur Balfour. At first Arthur was incredulous, but faced with the personal messages coming through he became fascinated and increasingly involved.

Moving conclusion

In 1929 a medium told Balfour, then an old man near death, of a beautiful lady she saw waiting for him in the next world. The lady was full of passionate tenderness and said: "tell him he gives me joy." Balfour seized the medium's hands fiercely, his eyes glittering. After that he was said to have welcomed death, knowing that the woman he had loved (who had been dead for over 50 years) would be waiting for him.

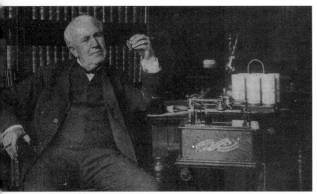

Thomas Alva Edison

STAYING ON THE LINE

Thomas Edison's parents believed in spiritualism, and he too was fascinated by the idea of life after death. He spent some years trying to develop a telephone that could be used between the dead and the living. In 1920 *American Magazine* printed the claim that Edison was at work on such an invention, and he publicly confirmed this was true a week later.

Telephone fault

Edison kept his machines secret until they were patented, so little is known about what he may have planned but never completed. However, in 1941 a blueprint was found in New York for a telephone to contact the dead, and this was alleged to be Edison's plan. It may well have been a fraud. In any case, a model was made from the designs, but unfortunately it didn't work.

Morbid receiver
Research by D. Scott Rogo and Raymond Bayless has led them to the conclusion that hundreds of telephone calls from the dead are received each year in America alone.

He went on to suggest that, if well-known composers had survived death, it should be simple for them to produce musical communications. Beethoven could supply a new symphony, or Wagner a new opera.

Clive-Ross issued his challenge in a comparatively obscure publication. A year later, and without knowledge of Clive-Ross's article, Rosemary Brown, a London housewife who had been psychic since childhood, began to write music in the styles of Bach, Beethoven, Brahms, Chopin, Debussy, Liszt, Rachmaninoff, and other composers. She says all of these works are written by the composers in the next world and then dictated to her at speed. Most communicate in English but "Liszt tends to go off into a stream of German when excited — or French." Her only musical training had been a few piano lessons. Some of the works are too difficult for her to play. Distinguished

> ## "It seems that their aim is not necessarily to transmit great music, but simply to prove their existence."

pianist John Lill is convinced that the compositions are genuine. He has said that some of Beethoven's spirit compositions are simplified, perhaps because Rosemary Brown is not always able to take down very complicated music. "Besides," he observes, "it seems to me that their [the spirit composers'] aim is not necessarily to try to transmit great music, but simply to prove their existence."

Luiz Antonio Gasparetto is to art what Rosemary Brown is to music.

The young Brazilian medium is a psychologist who produces works in the style of the old masters. His collection includes new Renoirs, Cezannes, and Picassos. Like Rosemary Brown, he says he sees and talks to dead artists.

The most famous Brazilian medium, however, is undoubtedly Francisco Candido (Chico) Xavier from the town of Pedro Leopoldo, in the state of Minas Gerais. Xavier is held in such high esteem in his country that he has even featured on a series of Brazilian postage stamps. Xavier spent at least five hours a day for 50 years allowing dead authors to write through him while in a trance. Having had only an elementary schooling, much of what he writes is beyond Xavier's understanding. He takes no money for his mediumship and the royalties from his books finance a welfare center.

Shared writing

One of Xavier's most impressive achievements as a medium is a work which seems to be yet another example of cross-correspondence. *Evolution in Two Worlds* was not dictated in the normal way. It came, one chapter at a time, in a form that made little sense. Only when the work was finished was Chico Xavier told by his spirit guide that he had been given *alternate* chapters. The missing sections had been dictated to another automatic writing medium, Dr. Waldo Vieira, who lived 250 miles away. It was the first of 17 books the two of them have produced in this way.

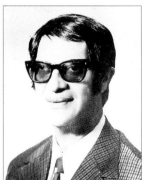

Chico Xavier
By the mid-1970's he had produced 130 books containing the works of 400 dead authors.

Are the works of the automatists a proof of contact between this

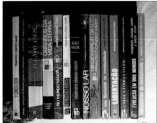

Automatic publications
Over three million copies of Xavier's books have been sold.

world and the next? And would such evidence ever stand up in a court of law? In fact, it has. In 1980 José Nunes was charged with killing his best friend Mauricio Henrique, at Goiania, in Brazil. The police refused to believe José's claim that the shooting was an accident, so his mother decided to ask Chico Xavier if he could contact Mauricio. Xavier did, and he attended José's trial to read the spirit message he had received by automatic writing. "José is not to blame," the dead friend reportedly declared. When the handwriting of the automatic writing script was compared with Mauricio's, they were found to be the same. As he gave his verdict on the case, Judge Orimar de Bastos told the

> ## "It is unprecedented for the victim, after his death, to give an account of his death."

hushed court that Chico Xavier was highly regarded for his honesty and would not make up such messages. "I am not a spiritualist," said the judge, "but I feel I have to give some credibility to this message — even though it is unprecedented for the victim, after his death, to give an account of his death. Mauricio's message backs up what José has told us. José Nunes is not guilty."

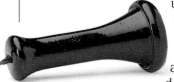

LINES OF COMMUNICATION

Communicating with the spirit world directly, rather than through a medium, has been the great dream of scientists and psychical researchers for decades.

THE INVENTOR OF the phonograph, Thomas A. Edison, and Guglielmo Marconi, inventor of the radio, both hoped to establish some form of electronic contact with the next world. Edison and Marconi didn't achieve their aim, but others claim to have succeeded. What is more, they say that anyone with a radio and a tape recorder (and a lot of patience) can receive voices from the next world. The electronic voice phenomenon (EVP) first gained public attention in 1959, when Friedrich Jürgenson, a Swede, announced that he had picked up the voice of his dead mother on a recording of bird calls in a forest. On hearing of Jürgenson's recordings, Dr. Konstantin Raudive, a Latvian-born psychologist living in Sweden, tried the same experiment, apparently with remarkable results.

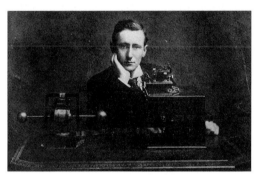

Guglielmo Marconi

What sounded like voices to Raudive and other researchers were dismissed by skeptics as just atmospheric buzzing. Often, Raudive could make sense of the voices only by assuming that the speaker was using three languages in a single sentence. He claimed to have recorded the voices of Churchill, Tolstoy, John F. Kennedy, Hitler, and Stalin.

Long-lost friends
More recently, D. Scott Rogo and Raymond Bayless have continued EVP research in the United States with experiments that have overcome some earlier criticisms. The scope of their investigations has broadened following reports of phone calls from the dead. Totally spontaneous messages have been received over the phone by people who say they recognized the voices of friends and relatives who had died.

In *Phone Calls From the Dead*, published in 1979, Rogo and Bayless reported their findings. One common feature of these calls

is that there is no click at the end of the message, as happens when someone hangs up normally. Most callers seem to be trying to make simple contact with the living, but sometimes an urgent message is delivered.

Rogo and Bayless were told one intriguing story by a well-known Hollywood actress who wanted to remain anonymous. As an eight-year-old child, she was at the home of a close friend of her mother's. It was Thanksgiving and there were a number of adults and children present. The friend's daughter had been killed in an automobile accident a few years previously. When the telephone rang, the actress answered the

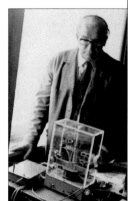

Konstantin Raudive
Dr. Raudive claimed that the so-called white noise between radio stations contained voices of the dead.

phone. A long-distance operator said she had a collect call for the mother from her daughter. The actress went to get the mother and remembers watching her as she took the phone. "She listened on the phone, turned absolutely white, and fainted." It appears that the dead daughter had spoken to her mother. No record of the call could be traced, and it was never charged for.

Hazy images
Klaus Schreiber, from West Germany, turned his basement into a laboratory for electronic contact with the dead. He started with tape recorders in 1982, then used video and television. Special amplifiers have helped Schreiber bring hazy shapes into focus as recognizable faces.

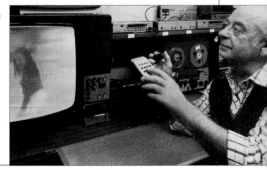

Art From The Past

"I don't really like working with Bach. He is very stern....When he comes to the house it's just for work, work, work....Like the others, Liszt brought him to the house the first time."
Rosemary Brown, *Unfinished Symphonies*

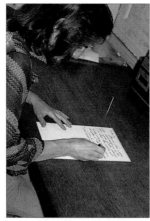

DO ARTISTIC GENIUSES continue to produce work after their deaths? A number of psychic painters, musicians, and writers claim that they are communicating new work by talents such as Picasso, Bach, and Jane Austen.

The suggestion is that some of the world's great creators are trying to prove their continuing existence by channeling work through certain selected "sensitives." Some of the resulting art is good in its own right, and much seems to reflect the style of well-known masters.

A link to the great artists

Englishman Matthew Manning began producing psychic art when he was a teenager in the early 1970's. His book *The Link* described his way of making contact. He merely sat quietly with pad and pen and concentrated on the artist's work. He did not enter a trance, but the pen just seemed to move, producing work in the dead artist's style. Picasso first came through in 1973 and Manning says his hand was moved with "excessive force." Paul Klee, Leonardo da Vinci, Albrecht Dürer, and Aubrey Beardsley are among the other artists whose styles are recognizable in Manning's collection.

A Brazilian trance artist, Luiz Antonio Gasparetto, appeared on television in 1978 and produced 21 new paintings in the styles of old masters. He accomplished this in a mere 75 minutes, often working with both hands simultaneously. New pictures in the styles of such masters as Renoir and Picasso seemed to appear magically. Gasparetto, a psychologist, claimed that he could not paint unless he went into a trance.

The art produced is often attractive, but the question remains: Are dead geniuses trying to perpetuate their creative powers — or are moderately clever people simply achieving fame and fortune by using the names and styles of the great?

Manning producing automatic writing

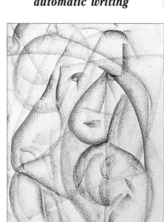

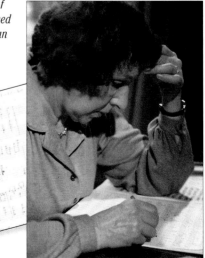

Demanding work
Manning felt ill while working on this sketch of a hanged man and wanted to stop, but felt compelled to finish by the anonymous contributor.

Exhausting genius
This painting in the style of Picasso came to Manning after the artist's death in 1973. Manning has said: "No other communicator tires me out as much as Picasso does. After only a few minutes, the time it takes him to do one drawing, I feel worn out and cannot continue for at least 24 hours."

In tune with the spirits
In her autobiographical book Unfinished Symphonies, *London housewife Rosemary Brown described how over 400 new compositions in the distinct styles of the masters were channeled through her. She claimed that she was visited by the spirit of Liszt when she was seven and that he promised to work through her as she became older. This manuscript shows a piece dictated to Rosemary Brown by Chopin. Her reflection of the nuances of the composers has convinced some people that more than imitation is involved.*

Polish composer Frédéric Chopin (1810-49)

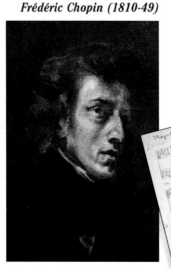

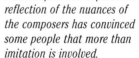

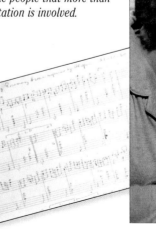

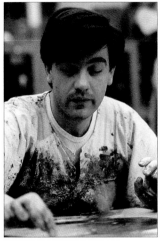

Working in the dark
Luiz Antonio Gasparetto produced most of his psychic paintings in just a few minutes, but some took several hours to complete. He normally worked in a trance in the dark or in very dim light.

The mark of an artist
Gasparetto's creations are sometimes signed — like this crayon drawing, which bears the signature of the French Impressionist painter Renoir.

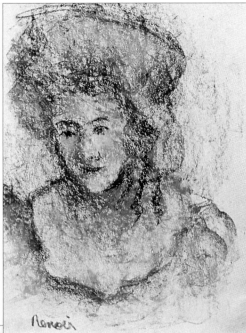

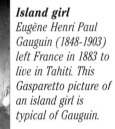

Vivid colors
Pierre Auguste Renoir (1841-1919) was especially renowned for his use of vivid pink and orange.

Island girl
Eugène Henri Paul Gauguin (1848-1903) left France in 1883 to live in Tahiti. This Gasparetto picture of an island girl is typical of Gauguin.

A Degas dancer
This painting of a dancer was produced by Gasparetto in the recognizable style of the French artist Edgar Degas (1834-1917).

Face value
Elongated faces were a feature of paintings by the Italian artist Amedeo Modigliani (1884-1920). This picture by Gasparetto (below) reflects the influence of Modigliani.

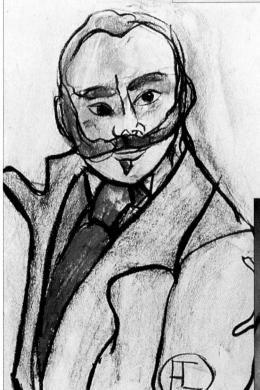

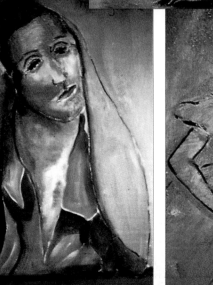

Familiar flourish
The characteristic style of the French painter Henri Toulouse-Lautrec (1864-1901), famous for his pictorial observations of Paris and its colorful characters, seems particularly familiar in this painting by Gasparetto.

Contemporary Channels

"Through my tears I saw what looked like a handful of gold and silver glitter sprinkled in a ray of sunshine. A very large entity was standing there....He looked at me with a beautiful smile and said, 'I am Ramtha, the enlightened one. I have come to help you over the ditch.' "
J. Z. Knight

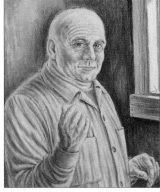

Visiting entity
Seth, painted by Jane Roberts's husband.

PSYCHIC EXPLOSION

Jane Roberts was one of the first and best-known channelers. A New York state would-be poet and novelist, she had her first psychic experience one evening in 1963: "A fantastic avalanche of new ideas burst into my head...some 100 pages flowed onto paper...."

A prolific partnership

Later in 1963, Roberts became aware that she had a "visiting entity" speaking through her. She and her husband, Robert F. Butts, became interested in the ouija board. With this they contacted a spirit called Frank Withers, a local resident who said he had died in 1942. Withers wanted to be known as Seth. Within a month Jane Roberts was going into trances and speaking for Seth. This contact continued for 21 years until Roberts died in 1984. She published five books channeled by Seth and two more books about her relationship with the spirit. The books encouraged New Agers in their interest in channeling.

Martian message
This alien communication was channeled through Hélène Smith in 1898.

THOUGH NOT A NEW phenomenon, channeling is enjoying unprecedented popularity as part of the New Age movement. The mechanics of channeling are similar to those of mediumship.

Mediums generally act as intermediaries for spirits trying to prove their earthly identities and their continuing existence in the next world. Channelers, on the other hand, allow themselves to be used by beings from other worlds, planets, dimensions, or even other levels of consciousness. Channelers are not concerned with trying to prove the communicators' identities. They say it is the *messages* that are important.

Out of this world

The history of channeling can be traced back to shamans in various ancient cultures who went into trances and were possessed by spirits. Such diverse authorities as the prophet Moses and the Oracle of Delphi could also be considered channelers. Emanuel Swedenborg (1688–1772), the Swedish seer and scientist, was probably the first modern channeler. In his book *Heaven and Hell*, Swedenborg claimed to visit the afterlife, as well as other planets. In *Concerning the Earths in Our Solar System* he described the inhabitants of Mars, Venus, and the Moon.

A Swiss medium, Catherine Elise Müller (who used the pseudonym Hélène Smith), claimed in 1894 that she too was in contact with Martians. She described the human, animal, and floral life on Mars, and spoke Martian. In 1899, Professor Theodore Flournoy, a sitter in her circle, disproved most of her supranormal claims in his book *From India to the Planet Mars*.

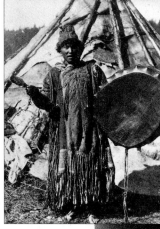

Siberian shaman

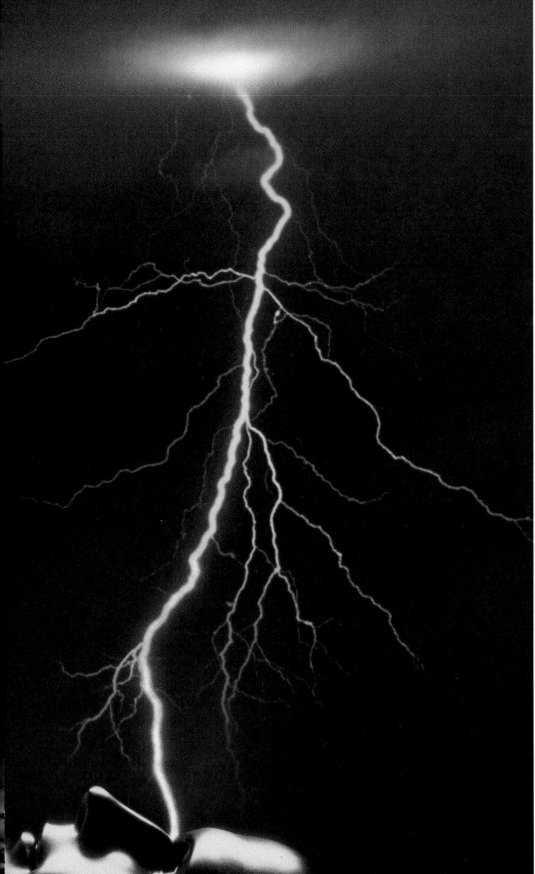

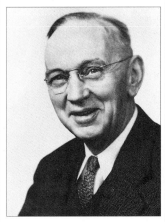

Psychic healer Edgar Cayce

WISH TO HELP OTHERS

Edgar Cayce was born in Hopkinsville, Kentucky, in 1877 and had his first psychic encounter in 1890 when the vision of a lovely woman granted him a single wish. He asked to be able to help others. Over a 40-year career Cayce published several books about his ability to heal and to see into the past and the future.

Systematic analysis

Cayce was one of the first trance mediums to have his words analyzed and catalogued in a systematic way. He founded the Association for Research and Enlightenment in Virginia Beach, Virginia, as an archive for his numerous readings. Although no spirits visited him, Cayce claimed to have tapped into a universal subconscious.

Key figure

Mediums today credit Cayce with being a key figure in the development of modern channeling. After Cayce's death in 1945, author Jess Stearn started to write his biography. As part of her research, Stearn approached a medium with a view to contacting Cayce. According to Stearn, Cayce announced that he would be guiding her hand, and the resulting book, *The Sleeping Prophet*, was written in only a few weeks. The volume sold millions of copies, and helped to establish the popularity of books by channelers.

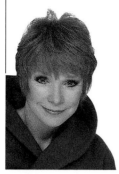

Shirley MacLaine

CELEBRITY ENDORSEMENT

In her bestselling books *Dancing in the Light* and *Out on a Limb*, actress Shirley MacLaine describes how experience with channelers has changed her life. "I found myself gently but firmly exposed to dimensions of time and space that heretofore, for me, belonged in science fiction or what I would describe as the occult. But it happened to me....What I learned as a result has enabled me to get on with my life as an almost transformed human being."

Gathering intelligence
Channelers, like mediums, try to link the living and the dead. But while mediums limit their contacts to the dead, channelers also connect with spirits in other forms — such as elves, dolphins, or even entities that have not lived on earth.

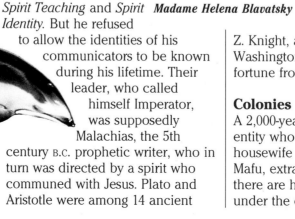

In more recent times a British cabdriver, George King, was one of the first to claim to be a channel for interplanetary entities. A voice told him in 1954: "Prepare yourself, you are to become the voice of Interplanetary Parliament." The subsequent trance messages from an alien being called Aetherius (from Venus) led to the founding of the Aetherius Society. Believers claim that Aetherius and other entities exist on the spiritual, astral planes of the planets, which is why our exploration of space has not detected them.

"Prepare yourself, you are to become the voice of Interplanetary Parliament."

Madame Helena Blavatsky, founder of the Theosophical Society, channeled *The Secret Doctrine* by direct astral access to two Tibetan mahatmas. And Edgar Cayce channeled his higher consciousness to give readings to 6,000 people over 43 years.

Spirit wisdom

Many spiritualist mediums are also known as channelers if they are the exclusive mouthpiece for entities whose purpose is to instill wisdom in those who listen. Rev. Stainton Moses, one of the most prominent spiritualists of the 19th century, received automatic writing scripts from a band of 49 spirits, which he published as *Spirit Teaching* and *Spirit Identity*. But he refused to allow the identities of his communicators to be known during his lifetime. Their leader, who called himself Imperator, was supposedly Malachias, the 5th century B.C. prophetic writer, who in turn was directed by a spirit who communed with Jesus. Plato and Aristotle were among 14 ancient

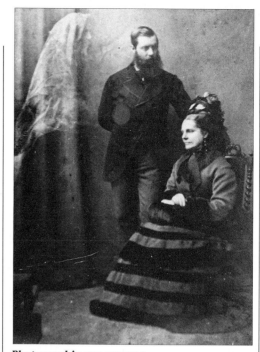

Photographic appearance
Rev. Stainton Moses and a fellow spiritualist pictured with a visitor from the spirit world.

philosophers and sages who also communicated through the reverend. More recently some spirit guides have been Native Americans. The teachings of Silver Birch, Red Cloud, and White Eagle have won them thousands of admirers. Some of these guides have discussed their lives on earth while others try to cloak their real identities in anonymity.

Today's channelers often produce entities who are far more colorful than their spiritualist counterparts. Ramtha, for example, who calls himself "the enlightened one," is said to be a 35,000-year-old warrior who once lived on Atlantis. He speaks through J. Z. Knight, a former housewife from Washington state who has made a fortune from her channeling enterprises.

Madame Helena Blavatsky

Colonies under earth

A 2,000-year-old man named Mafu is the entity who speaks through California housewife Penny Torres. According to Mafu, extraterrestrials live among us and there are humanoid colonies living under the earth.

Equally famous as a communicator is Seth, who spoke through the trance mediumship of Jane Roberts from 1963 until her death in 1984. The first book of his teachings was entitled *The Seth Material*, followed by *Seth Speaks: The Eternal Validity of the Soul*.

The themes expressed by channelers are much the same. You create and make your own path in life. You already have the knowledge necessary to lead a wise life, and channelers only help to activate it.

Jach Pursel, a former Florida insurance supervisor, claims that in 1984 he was entered by a being called Lazaris. Pursel now spends up to 40 hours a week in an unconscious state while Lazaris speaks through him. "Lazaris tells us how to change our lives and then teaches us specific techniques to accomplish the change," explains Pursel. Lazaris spreads his teachings by means of private readings, weekend workshops, and public talks, all of which are administered by Pursel's corporation, Concept: Synergy, which operates out of Fairfax, California.

The obscure origins attributed to channeled entities make it difficult for skeptics to challenge them scientifically. When Emmanuel, who speaks through Pat Radagast, was asked about himself,

> ### "Rather than attempt to understand who I am, allow whatever experience comes to you to be honored."

the response was typical: "Rather than attempt to understand who I am, allow whatever experience comes to you to be honored." He said that it does not matter whether he is another being or simply a deeper part of the channeler, because, in the end, "the truth and the

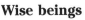

intuitive validity of what Emmanuel says is what really matters."

Sarah Grey Thomason, a professor of linguistics at the University of Pittsburgh, has investigated the claims of various channelers and found that language can be useful in determining the authenticity of historical facts. For example, both Ramtha and Mafu are said to speak in a vaguely British accent — highly unusual, given their otherworldly origins. Prof. Thomason also analyzed a recording of an entity named Matthew, whom his channeler, Marjorie Turcott, described as a poor, blind fiddle-player from early 16th-century Scotland. After describing a variety of linguistic errors (*Skeptical Inquirer*, Summer 1989), Prof. Thomason says that Matthew's accent sounds as if it were being faked

Indian influence
This painting shows "Skiwaukie," spirit guide to medium Mary Hollis-Billing.

by someone unfamiliar with Scots English. However, after she had listened "to his audience's respectful reception to Matthew's pronouncements on the Bermuda Triangle, the civilization inside the hollow earth, UFO's, and psychic surgery...." Prof. Thomason concluded that the authenticity of an accent is not important to Matthew's followers.

Wise beings

In the end, it may not be the authenticity of any spirit link that really matters. As channelers insist, it is the message that counts. Kathryn Ridall, the author of *Channeling: How to Reach Out to Your Spirit Guides*, admits in her introduction: "Ultimately we can never know for sure whether channeling is a complete fabrication of our own minds....But if we have invented all these channelings, the human mind has an amazing capacity to access wisdom far beyond our conscious knowledge. And if we have not made it up, then the universe is full of many wise beings who love us and want to help us."

AGE OF ENLIGHTENMENT

A woman living near Seattle, Washington, J. Z. Knight, claims that she was first visited by "the enlightened one," a 35,000-year-old male spirit named Ramtha, in 1977. Believers have flocked to her sessions, and Knight says she has earned millions of dollars from the phenomenon.

In 1986 *Newsweek* described a typical session: "Knight induces a semiconscious state, shakes, then goes limp. Reanimating as Ramtha, Knight walks through the audience speaking in a low,

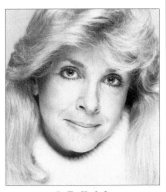

J. Z. Knight

rhythmic voice. She says the transformation is so complete that she must later hear a recording to discover what Ramtha said."

In his book *Channeling*, Jon Klimo discussed the possibility that channels may "burn out," and by the 1980's some critics were saying that whatever energy had been coming through J. Z. Knight had indeed departed.

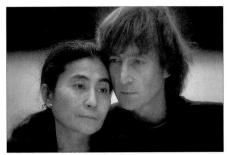

John Lennon and Yoko Ono
Some channelers claim to be amplifying the spirits of dead stars. California channeler William Tenuto says he is speaking as the "voice" of John Lennon, who was murdered in 1980.

DO NOT DISTURB

In the 1830's, before he became a well-known writer, Nathaniel Hawthorne (1804–64) went to Boston's Athenaeum library each day to work for a few hours. Another regular visitor was Rev. Doctor Harris, an old clergyman who sat in a chair by the fireplace, reading newspapers.

Clerical presence

Hawthorne never spoke to Harris but noted his presence. It came as a great surprise when a friend told Hawthorne that Rev. Harris had been a regular visitor to the library, but that the old man had died a while ago.

On subsequent visits to the library, Hawthorne continued to see the clergyman sitting by the fireplace. Hawthorne did not try to touch the figure or establish contact.

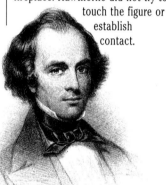

Nathaniel Hawthorne

As Hawthorne said: "Perhaps I was loath to destroy the illusion, and to rob myself of so good a ghost story, which might have been explained in some very commonplace way."

Feeling foolish

The writer also confessed that he hesitated to try to talk to what might have looked like an empty chair to other people: "What an absurd figure I would have made."

One day, some months after learning that the old man was dead, Hawthorne went into the Athenaeum and saw that the chair by the fireplace was now empty. He never saw Harris again.

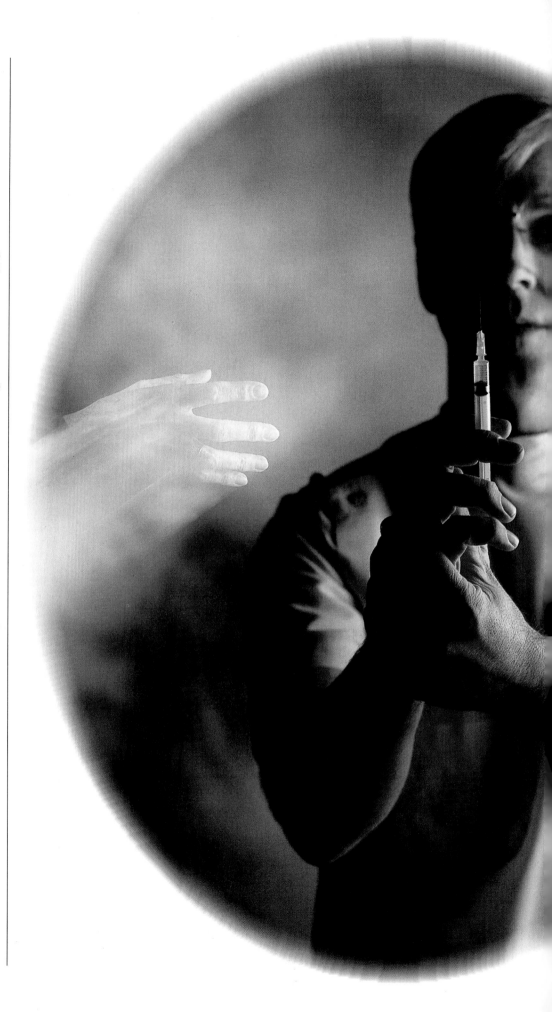

FANTASTIC VISIONS

Surveys show that thousands of people have seen apparitions. They may be suffering from hallucinations, but many are sure that these visitors come from the past, the future, or from beyond the grave.

A DENTIST IN BUTTE, Montana, was about to inject a patient with anesthetic before extracting a tooth when a strange feeling made him withdraw the needle before injecting. The troubled dentist retreated into his laboratory, where a vision of his mother appeared to him, warning that the patient wanted to die and hoped to receive a fatal dose of the painkiller. In effect, the patient would be committing suicide, but the dentist would bear the blame and the patient's family would not lose the life insurance benefit. The dentist went back to the patient and asked about any problems with the anesthetic being used. The patient then admitted that a previous injection had caused him to black out and that it had taken doctors several hours to bring him back to full consciousness again.

Familiar visitors

History and folklore are full of tales of apparitions and ghostly beings. They appear to be of the everyday world but exhibit otherworldly characteristics, such as gradually fading from sight or passing through solid objects. Sometimes the vision is of a recognizable person, but not always. The apparitions may manifest for an obvious purpose, such as issuing a warning or giving help. But in some cases the reason for the appearance is not clear. Whether they comfort or terrify, apparitions are very real to those who believe they have seen them.

First president
Professor Henry Sidgwick, president of the SPR 1882-84.

International claims

One of the first major surveys carried out by the Society for Psychical Research (SPR) was the 1889 Census of Hallucinations. This was undertaken in conjunction with the International Congress on Experimental Psychology. Thousands of people in different countries were asked: "Have you ever, when believing yourself to be completely awake, had a vivid impression of seeing or being touched by a living being or inanimate object, or of hearing a voice — which impression, so far as you could discover, was not due to any external cause?"

Over 17,000 replies were received from Austria, Brazil, France, Germany, Italy, Russia, and Britain. Nearly 10 percent of those polled claimed that they had seen or otherwise sensed an apparition.

UNBIASED RESEARCH

In the mid-1800's paranormal activities were rarely out of the news. Believers in the new religion of spiritualism said that they were convinced of the existence of life after death, because they had spoken to the dead through the psychic powers of mediums. By the late 1870's spiritualism had spread from America to England, and it was with the intention of providing unbiased and informed research into the paranormal that a number of scholars and scientists decided to form the Society of Psychical Research (SPR) in London, in February 1882.

Eminent scientists

Sir William Barrett, professor of psychics at the Royal College of Science in Dublin, called the meeting that established the SPR. The first president of the society was Cambridge professor of classics, Henry Sidgwick, one of many eminent intellectuals in the 18-member founding council. In 1885, Sir William Barrett helped to set up the American Society of Psychical Research (ASPR).

A modern approach

The popularity of the paranormal, spurred on by famous mediums and their dramatic séances, reached its peak between the two world wars. By the 1940's the SPR, influenced by the pioneering work of Dr. J. B. Rhine in the U.S., was turning its attentions toward research into extrasensory perception (ESP). Since the 1960's the society has concentrated on developing increasingly sophisticated testing equipment. To this day the society continues to take a scientific approach to the paranormal, and as an organization it still holds no overall opinion regarding psychic phenomena.

A SENSE OF THE UNREAL

A hallucination is a perception (such as hearing voices or seeing faces) that has no external stimulus. It is different from an illusion, which is the misinterpretation of a real stimulus.

Hearing things

Hallucinations can occur as a result of physical or mental disorders. Schizophrenics often hear voices or experience touch and taste hallucinations. People with temporal lobe epilepsy have been known to imagine smells. A whole range of temporary hallucinations are also brought on as a result of sensory deprivation or immense physical stress.

Withdrawal symptoms

Visual hallucinations are frequent during states of delirium caused by a physical illness, such as pneumonia. Hallucinations may also occur when chronic alcoholics quit drinking. Without their regular intake of alcohol, alcoholics suffer from *delirium tremens*. This is a state of extreme confusion accompanied by trembling, together with vivid hallucinations that often feature insects — particularly spiders.

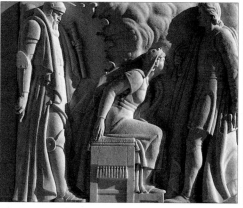

Shakespeare's ghosts
Shakespeare took ghosts seriously and his phantom characters seem very real. This sculpted relief shows a scene from Hamlet, *in which the ghost of Hamlet's father is fully armed and armored and "doom'd for a certain term to walk the night...."*

A similar type of survey was tried in Los Angeles in the 1980's by psychologist Julian Burton. In his study about half of the respondents claimed to have had some contact with the dead or other psychical experience. The 1889 census had been conducted among the general population, but Burton started by polling members of psychic study groups. The rate of positive response stayed just as high when psychology students at three Los Angeles colleges were questioned. Further studies among a more general population also produced a high percentage of positive replies.

Maternal influence

Burton was prompted to carry out his research by an experience he had in 1980. One evening when he went into his kitchen he met an apparition of his mother, who had died seven years earlier. She seemed to be wearing a diaphanous pale blue gown trimmed with feathers, which Burton had not seen before. When he rang his sister the next day, she recalled shopping with their mother a few weeks before her death. Strangely, their mother had admired a gown just like the one he had seen her wearing. In Burton's case it wasn't clear why

his mother had appeared to him. Other apparitions of the dead seem meant to comfort the living. In 1983, Kalis Osis (who was director of research at the American Society for Psychical Research from 1962 to 1975) studied a case that was a good example of the dead returning to reassure those left behind.

Osis reported that a 36-year-old businessman had been killed when the small airplane he was flying across the southern U.S. crashed. His wife was devastated. The couple's young son had died shortly before the crash, and the double tragedy left her inconsolable.

One night the unhappy woman woke to see her dead husband and baby son standing at the foot of the bed, holding hands. She said they seemed very happy to have found each other — and this gave her some comfort. "They were solid. There was grayness around, like a gray cloud...mist in the whole room." The

> ## "They were solid. There was grayness around ...mist in the whole room."

vision lasted for about 15 seconds and then simply faded out.

The woman said she had no belief in an afterlife until this experience. "If someone had told me about an experience like I had, I would think that person belonged in an institution."

Another skeptic who found himself receiving an apparition was Rev. Russell H. Conwell, a distinguished clergyman and founder of Temple University in Philadelphia. In the early 1900's, soon after his wife's death, Rev. Conwell saw a vision of her every morning at the foot of his bed. The apparition initially surprised him but seemed extremely real and even talked with him. Rev. Conwell decided to put it to several tests. First, the vision correctly revealed where his army discharge papers were kept. Second, he asked his housemaid to hide a pen and the next day the apparition correctly told him where it was hidden.

The clergyman was amazed. When he said one day to the vision, "I know you aren't really there," the apparition cheerfully replied, "Oh, but I am...."

RUTH AND REALITY

By definition, hallucinations have no reality. They are merely constructed by a disordered brain. This is the standard view, but the story of one psychiatric patient raises intriguing questions. Is it possible for hallucinations to become apparitions visible to others, real entities with a life of their own?

IN THE LATE 1970's Ruth, a 25-year-old American living in London, went to psychiatrist Dr. Morton Schatzman for help in overcoming her agoraphobia, or fear of going out in public. It soon became clear to Dr. Schatzman that Ruth's real problem was fear of the hallucinations she had been having of her father, who had abused her sexually as a child. Ruth's hallucinations were extremely strong and realistic: "I can count his teeth," said Ruth. "I can smell him." Ruth lived in terror of these manifestations, which appeared without warning. Schatzman suggested that she confront the matter head-on by conjuring up the images of her father, in order to banish them. This took a great deal of time and courage, but eventually she was able to do it.

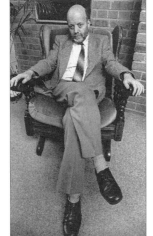

Dr. Morton Schatzman

Imagined reality

Schatzman discovered that Ruth's ability to create hallucinations had wider implications. He knew that Ruth was not insane — but she possessed an astonishing capacity to create images that were completely real to her.

In one experiment Ruth proved she could hallucinate Dr. Schatzman while the doctor sat elsewhere. Monitoring equipment showed that she was actually "seeing" a figure.

Ruth then experimented by deliberately hallucinating her husband while he was away on business. When driving on her own, she would sometimes put an apparition on the seat beside her, for company. But the case's most significant aspect was that her creations were seen by someone else.

A shared experience

While visiting her family in the U.S., Ruth made an apparition of her husband Paul sitting behind the steering wheel of her car. She told her father to look in the car and tell her what he saw. "Oh yeah," he said, "It looks like a ghost sitting in there. Isn't that the damndest thing? It looks like a man, just like Paul...."

On another occasion, Ruth created an apparition of herself sitting on the sofa while the real Ruth sat on a chair out of the way by the front door. Her husband Paul reacted as if he had seen a ghost. "You were just sitting on the sofa. How did you get over to that chair?" he said. Ruth pointed out that she had been sitting on the chair the whole time and that she hadn't been near the sofa at all.

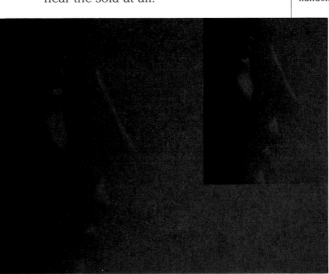

WHAT DID RUTH SEE?

Researchers have found that it is possible to register the presence of hallucinations by using an electroencephalogram (EEG) to monitor the brain's activity. An EEG records the electrical impulses generated by the brain.

Regular patterns

EEG subjects produce characteristic brain wave patterns in response to various conditions, such as resting with their eyes open or shut, or looking at a flashing light. If a subject's EEG readings indicate that he or she is responding to an external stimulus when one does not exist, this indicates that they are hallucinating.

Real entities

The results of EEG tests carried out on Ruth showed that her hallucinations evoked real, physical responses. Psychiatrist Dr. Morton Schatzman raised the query: "Could the entities Ruth allegedly saw and heard be real in some sense?"

PHANTOM CREW

In December 1972 an Eastern Airlines Tri-Star, flight 401, crashed into a Florida swamp. Among the 101 people killed were the pilot, Bob Loft, and the flight engineer, Don Repo. After the accident these two men were "seen" on over 20 occasions by crew on other Eastern Tri-Stars — especially those planes fitted with salvaged parts from the wreck.

Familiar faces

The apparitions were reported by people who had known the men and also by others who later recognized the faces from photographs. The story was well known in the airline world, and an account appeared in a 1974 newsletter of the U.S. Flight Safety Foundation.

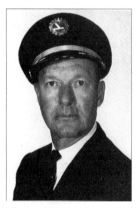

*Flight 401 pilot,
Bob Loft*

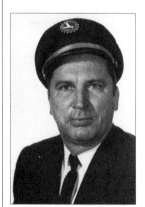

*Flight engineer, Second
Officer Don Repo*

While apparitions are commonly of people that are known and loved, sometimes the vision is not recognizable. In 1950, staff members from the American and British embassies in Oslo, Norway, went skiing outside the city. One of the Americans and a British couple exchanged remarks with a woman dressed in a herringbone tweed suit like those worn at the end of the 19th century. In an angry voice with a Scottish accent, the woman accused the skiers of trespassing. They apologized, and hastened away.

The diplomats were curious to know the woman's identity. When they made inquiries they discovered that a young couple owned the land they had been skiing on. The farm had been in the family for generations. Although there was no old woman currently living there, the present farmer's great-grandfather had married a Scottish girl.

"It was the most vivid experience, and I can recall it all in enormous detail. There is just no way it was a dream."

The skiers were sure they had seen "the girl from Scotland."

Children are often thought to be more psychically aware than adults, and many sightings of apparitions are reported by young people. One day in the late 1950's, eight-year-old Lee Stanton of York, England, was in bed recovering from flu. Suddenly an unfamiliar man appeared in the doorway.

"He was very gaunt and white-faced," says Lee, "with a handlebar mustache and a flat cap and muffler. I couldn't possibly see his feet, yet I could tell you that he was wearing very clumsy, cheap boots. He seemed to make up his mind about something and shambled off across the landing. It was the most vivid experience, and I can recall it all in enormous detail. There is just no way it was a dream."

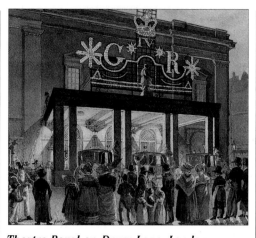

Theatre Royal on Drury Lane, London
The Theatre Royal supposedly harbors a number of apparitions. One is an Irish actor who killed another actor in 1735. The best-known ghost in the theater is called the Man in Gray. This young man wears an 18th-century riding cloak, boots, a three-sided hat, and carries a sword.

The man Lee saw may have been the ghost of her grandfather who used to live in the house. She had never met her grandfather or seen a photograph of him, and yet the description she gave fitted him perfectly.

Parapsychologist Dr. Ernesto Spinelli has shown that the younger the child, the higher its capacity to score well in ESP tests. This may explain the stories that children tell of imaginary playmates that their parents cannot see.

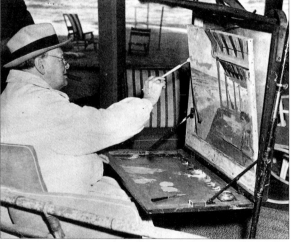

Father and son
People as rational and respectable as Winston Churchill have claimed to see apparitions. Churchill was painting in his studio, copying a portrait of his dead father, when his father appeared sitting in a leather chair nearby. Churchill said they had a good discussion about political events and changes over the previous few decades.

GHOSTS AND TIMESLIPS

Many ghost stories have an element of the timeslip, in which subjects appear to step into the past. Do these people then appear as ghosts from the future, capable of startling humans who lived long ago?

A CLASSIC STORY about an apparent timeslip involved a young workman named Martindale who was employed on renovations in the cellars of the Treasurer's House in York, England, in the 1960's. Alone at lunchtime, the boy was alarmed to hear a distant bugle, which seemed to be coming nearer. Before his horrified eyes, a group of tattered and fatigued Roman soldiers marched through the vaults.

Treasurer's House, York

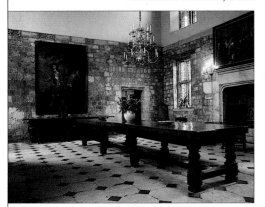

Viking invaders
In the area where the Whites saw the mysterious crowd of figures, there used to be a number of Roman camps. The same area was later occupied by invading Vikings who set up winter camps in the late 10th century. The Vikings used the island as a base from which to attack the mainland. The style of dress described by the Whites is more Viking than Roman.

Investigation showed that there was a Roman road under the floor of the house, exactly where Martindale had seen the soldiers. The ghostly crew had not taken any notice of him, so it seems that this timeslip may have been a historic event being replayed.

A timely meeting
Dr. and Mrs. White of the Isle of Wight report a similar timeslip experience. While driving slowly across the island one evening in January 1969, the couple became aware of unexplained lights, noises, and shadowy running figures. Slowing down almost to a complete stop, the Whites found themselves in the middle of a crowd of men carrying torches and wearing rough leather jerkins and broad belts in medieval style. The couple had the sensation that they were in the aftermath of a historic battle. One of the running men stopped and stared in horror through their windshield before dashing off into the gloom. The couple were sure that he had seen them. Then the whole vision faded.

Did the Whites figure in some breathless tale told over the fire centuries ago? Did they become the fairy folk who arrived after the battle in their strange chariot? We will never know. Perhaps strange-looking visitors, widely believed to be from outer space, are simply humans from the future.

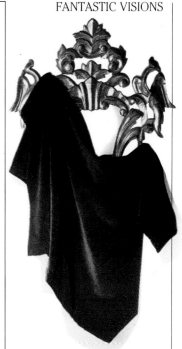

LIVING APPARITIONS
Visions are usually associated with the dead, but phantoms of the living have also been reported. The vision may be of another living person or even of oneself.

Departing soul
People in many parts of the world believe that if they see their own double, their soul has left the body and death is imminent. The ancient Greeks feared seeing their reflection in water, as the soul might become trapped there. Zulu people in southern Africa still hold this belief.

Mirror image
Some superstitions about mirrors are rooted in a fear that the "double" represents a bad omen. Many people believe that mirrors should be covered in a house where someone has just died. They warn against gazing in a mirror in the room where a corpse lies — as this could be fatal. Covering mirrors also prevents the dead person's soul from being trapped in the glass. A sick-room mirror should also be covered, as a weakened soul that leaves the body and becomes trapped in the glass might not have the strength to return, in which case the invalid will die.

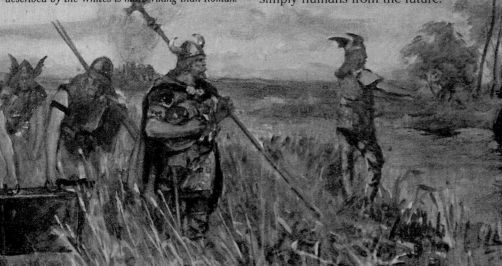

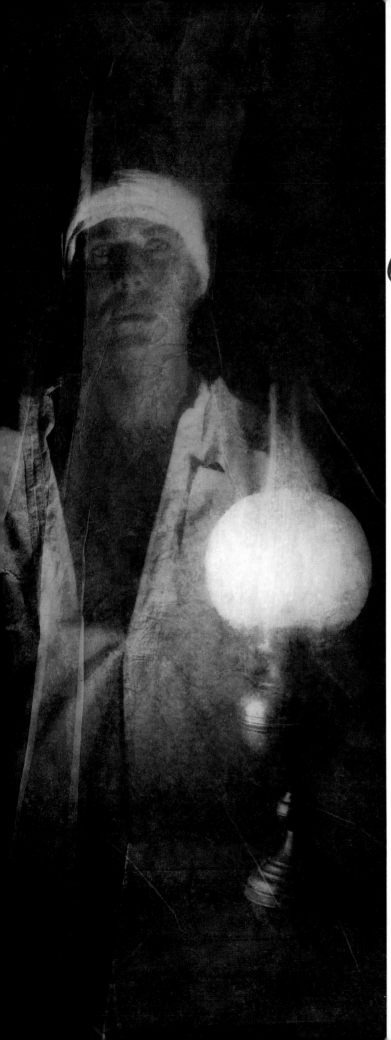

THE LAST FAREWELL

There are many cases on record of "crisis apparitions." A loved one unexpectedly appears and then disappears in a ghostly fashion — and is later found to have suffered a trauma or died around the time of the sighting.

ONE NIGHT IN JANUARY 1856, Mrs. Anne Collyer of Camden, New Jersey, awoke and was amazed to "see" her son Joseph standing in the doorway of her bedroom. It was extremely unlikely for him to be there, as he was the captain of a steamboat on the Mississippi River, over 1,000 miles away.

Mrs. Collyer was distraught to see her son with his face and head disfigured and wrapped in a bandage. The next morning, when she told her family what she had seen, they disregarded the vision as a bad dream.

Nearly two weeks later news arrived that Captain Collyer had died in a steamboat collision. His skull had been split as the ship's mast fell on him. His death occurred at approximately the time his mother saw the apparition of her distressed son.

His death occurred at approximately the time his mother saw the apparition.

The Society for Psychical Research found this case especially interesting. There was independent testimony from Mrs. Collyer's husband and daughters. An additional detail was striking. Anne Collyer reported to her family that she had seen her son in a soiled white nightshirt — and he died in a shirt exactly like the one she described.

Time of death
In 1886, researchers for the SPR published a 1,400-page survey called *Phantasms of the Living*. Of more than 700 cases described, over half included phantom appearances or impressions coinciding with death or another critical moment in a person's life. One of the authors, Edmund Gurney, wrote that they were "struck with the predominance of alleged apparitions at or near the moment of death...."

American playwright David Belasco has said he was prompted to write about the dead returning because of an experience he had involving his mother. Belasco was sleeping in New York when he woke and saw her in the room. This was quite a surprise, as she lived in San Francisco. Belasco's mother stood by him, smiling and calling "Davy, Davy, Davy." She told him not to be sad, as she was happy. The apparition then vanished.

Belasco felt certain that this meant his mother was dead. He contacted his family, and a telegram confirming her death arrived a few hours later. His mother had died at the time he had seen her in his room. Just before she died, she reportedly smiled and called out, "Davy, Davy, Davy."

The First World War, with its immense carnage involving millions of ordinary men and women, gave rise to a number of similar stories. A typical tale is that of the woman who, while working in her kitchen, heard footsteps in the hall. On going to investigate, she discovered her brother, whom she believed to be fighting in the trenches. He was staggering in a dazed condition, covered in mud, and white with shock. "Get me a cup of tea, Maude," he muttered. Hurriedly, his sister went into the kitchen to make some tea. When she returned to the hall, there was no one there. Her brother had disappeared. News came later that he had been killed in action at the time he had appeared to her.

Disturbed vision
Distressing apparitions cannot be explained away as wishful thinking. If Maude's vision had been a hopeful fantasy, her brother would have appeared well and happy to see her.

There could be another explanation: In the split second in which the soldier found himself losing consciousness, he projected himself to his home and his sister for comfort. This might explain his battledress and shell-shocked condition. It could be that when consciousness withdrew from his body to enter some after-death state, his apparition faded.

Observers of the "death coincidence," as the phenomenon is sometimes known, often see their loved ones as they actually are at the point of death. One father saw his son, a soldier, kneeling down. It was discovered later that the son's body was found in that position. His body had been propped up by the weight of other corpses. Another apparition was seen with a red spot in the middle of his forehead, exactly where the fatal bullet entered his body.

The debate about crisis and other apparitions continues. Do these phantoms take up real space or are they only hallucinations in the minds of the perceivers? Both Frederic Myers and Edmund Gurney of the SPR thought apparitions were explained by telepathy.

In the 1950's Dr. Hornell Hart of Duke University, North Carolina, rejected these earlier ideas. He suggested that apparitions had some real, independent existence and were involved with objects and people in the same way as a living person. Hart believed that apparitions were some kind of "soul body" that could be freed from the

---

Are people less willing to admit to seeing apparitions in our modern, scientific age?

---

physical body at death or during life. Dr. Louisa Rhine, who gathered the largest collection of hallucination experiences on record in the United States, thought differently. She regarded apparitions as a kind of ESP hallucination, existing only in the mind.

Fewer apparitions seem to be reported now than in years past. Are people less willing to admit to seeing apparitions in our modern scientific age — or could there be other explanations? Dr. Ian Stevenson of the University of Virginia Medical School has suggested that the great speed and ease of modern communications may be a factor. In many historical cases, people had not seen or spoken to their loved ones for months or years, and were desperate to make contact, by any means possible or impossible.

Some incidents for which "hallucination" or "telepathy" are unlikely explanations, offer striking support for the reality of apparitions. The following example is typical of the real experiences that have happened to ordinary people.

New colleague
In the mid-1950's an Englishwoman, Joan D., was working in an office in central London. A new woman joined the company and an unusual conversation took place between them a few days later. "Have you just lost someone in your family?" the new woman inquired. Joan looked surprised and replied that her father had indeed died very recently. "Did he have a gray-and-white Harris tweed jacket with leather patches on the elbows, leather on the cuffs of the sleeves, a gray cardigan...?" The woman went on to describe her colleague's father in great detail.

Watch over you
Joan sat down, somewhat stunned at how this new person in the office could know so much about her father. The woman then explained in a kind voice: "I'm a medium. I just wanted to let you know that your father was standing beside you a short while ago watching you work. He looked very happy."

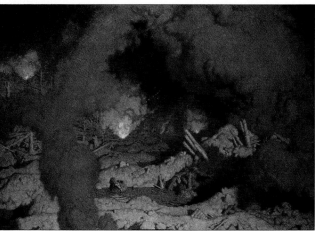

Time of crisis
The nightmarish conditions in the trenches during the First World War resulted in a horrific number of fatalities. During times of war, reports of crisis apparitions rise dramatically.

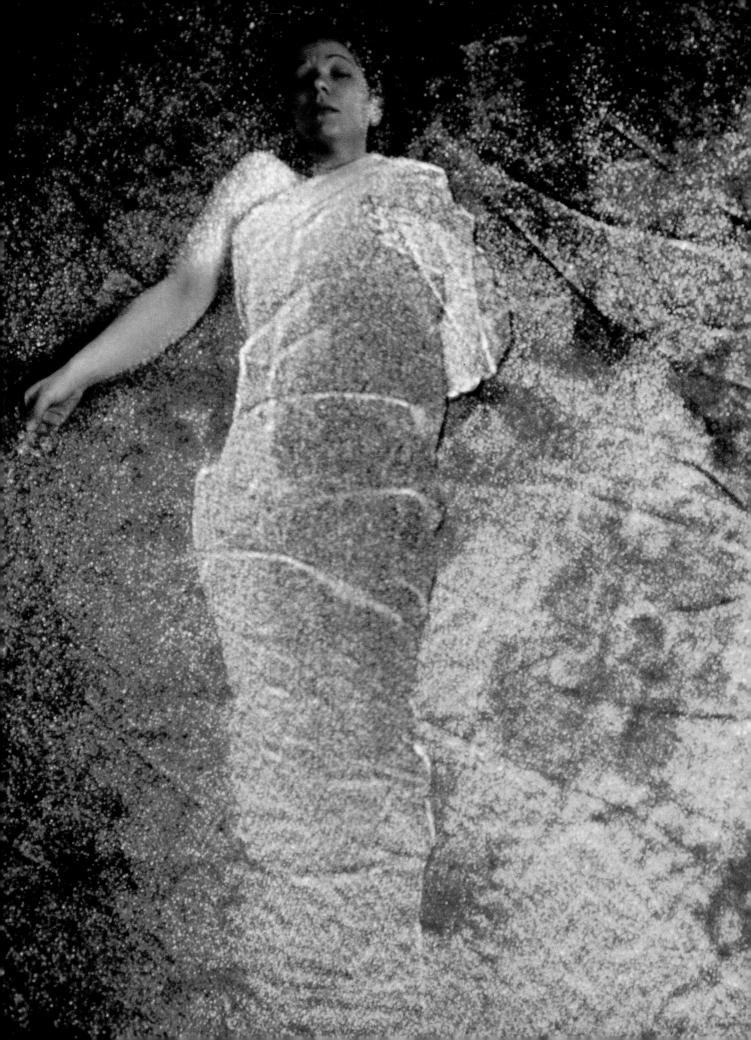

CHAPTER FOUR

DEATH: THE ENIGMA

One certainty for all humans is death. We die, decompose, and eventually become dust. Yet even in this process there are strange anomalies. In the amazing phenomenon of incorruptibility, dead bodies do not rot but may actually gain a beauty and radiance not possessed in life.

The Polish saint Andrew Bobola was martyred by the Cossacks in 1657. He was beaten savagely, tied to a horse, and then dragged for miles across rough, stony ground. Half his face was torn off, along with one of his limbs. His tormentors then killed him with a sword and buried him hastily in a churchyard in Pinsk. When St. Andrew was dug up 40 years later, his body was intact apart from the injuries — and

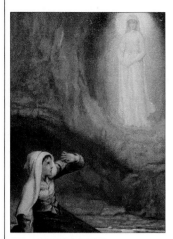

ST. BERNADETTE

The most famous incorruptible is St. Bernadette, a French peasant girl born Bernadette Soubirous. Her visions of the Virgin Mary established her hometown of Lourdes as a world center of pilgrimage. She died in 1879 at the age of 35, but her appearance today is said to be as fresh and lifelike as that of a sleeping girl. According to church authorities only a thin layer of wax covers her face to prevent discoloration.

A lasting vision

When St. Bernadette was exhumed in 1909, an eyewitness reported: "Not the least trace of corruption nor any bad odor could be perceived in the corpse of our beloved sister. Even the habit in which she was buried was intact. Her face was somewhat brown, the eyes slightly sunken and she seemed to be sleeping."

In public view

St. Bernadette's body is kept in a glass coffin in a chapel at Nevers, France. She is seen by thousands of pilgrims every year.

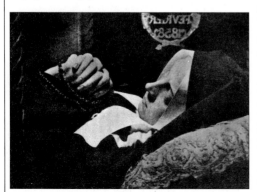

this despite being buried with gaping wounds, and decaying corpses all around him. Over the centuries St. Andrew was examined by doctors many times and in 1917 his still well-preserved body was put on public display.

St. Andrew's case is an example of the miracle of incorruptibility, by which the bodies of some saints have defied all natural laws, remaining intact and sweet-smelling long after death. References to an "odor of sanctity" appeared as early as A.D. 155, in a letter from the Christians of Smyrna describing

Restored in death

The incorrupt body of St. Teresa Margaret of the Sacred Heart is still on view in Florence, Italy. Disfigured by illness during her life, her body lost all signs of imperfection within two days of her death.

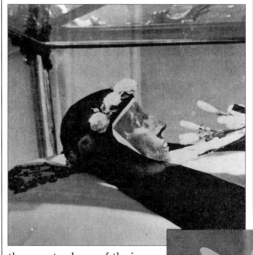

the martyrdom of their holy bishop, St. Polycarp: "We perceived such a fragrant smell, as if it were the wafted odor of frankincense."

The Incorruptibles, published in 1977, was written by Joan Cruz, a housewife from New Orleans. She cites 102 cases and speculates that there may be many more incorrupted Catholic saints lying undiscovered.

The body of the blessed Maria Anna Ladroni, who died in 1624, is said to have defied any decay. During the process of her beatification in 1731, an autopsy was ordered, at which 11 doctors were

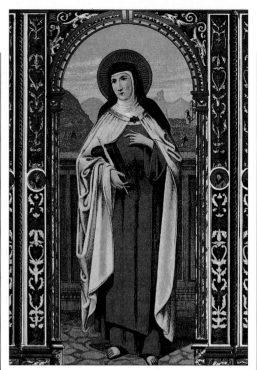

St. Teresa of Ávila

present. Deep incisions were made in several parts of the flesh. Her body was carefully examined to establish if any embalming fluids had been used to preserve it. No such substances were found, yet all her internal organs were discovered to be moist and completely intact. Her body had a fragrance that grew stronger and sweeter as the mystified surgeons examined it.

Telltale fragrance

The puzzle of incorruption is heightened by the fact that many saints met their deaths by violence or suffered such illnesses as cancer. Decomposition is likely to occur more quickly in bodies that have received severe injuries or suffered from wasting diseases. St. Teresa Margaret of the Sacred Heart (1747-70), suffered from a gangrenous disease involving the death and decay of tissues. This reduced her body to a grotesquely swollen, purple mass. However, two days after her death on March 7, 1770, the swelling and discoloration disappeared. She was left beautifully fresh and enveloped in the telltale fragrance of true incorruptibility. Her body can be viewed today, lying on show in a glass coffin in the chapel of the Monastery of St. Teresa in Florence, Italy. Dehydration

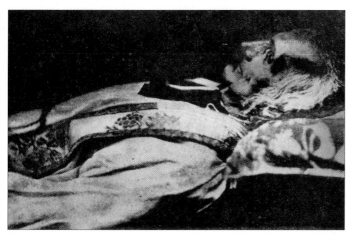

The Curé of Ars, France
St. Jean Baptiste Marie Vianney was a parish priest in Ars. His spiritual advice was much in demand during his life. Following his death in 1859, he continued to give inspiration – as an incorruptible.

has caused her skin to become very dark and leathery but she is still perfectly incorrupt.

Sometimes the conditions of a burial site have been so damp that clothes have rotted while the corpse has remained whole. This happened in the cases of such incorruptibles as St. Teresa of Ávila, St. Catherine Labouré, and Sts. Catherine of Genoa and Siena.

"If I was the murderer, then shall the good Lord never let my body rot."

Incorruptibility is seen generally by the religious as a divine favor bestowed on the truly devout. However, it has also affected some evil individuals.

Christian Kahlbutz, a 17th-century German knight, was certainly no saint. Despite being a hero on the battlefield, he was a tyrannical despot at home. He insisted on claiming the right to sleep with the brides of his vassals on their wedding nights. In addition to his 11 legitimate offspring, he is said to have fathered 30 children out of wedlock. When one vassal's bride refused his advances, he took revenge by killing her betrothed. An attempt was made to bring Kahlbutz to court, but he was protected by his power and position. He is said to have declared: "If I was the murderer, then shall the good Lord

never let my body rot." It appears that the Lord may have been listening. Kahlbutz died in 1707, but when his coffin was opened 90 years later, his body was found to be intact. Over a century and a half later, the dehydrated, leathery corpse was put on display as a public attraction in the tiny village of Kampehl near Berlin, during the 1936 Olympic Games.

Incorruptibility does not depend on the body being kept whole. St. Catherine of Siena had been a stigmatic during her life. On her death in 1380, the marks of Christ's Passion were visible on her hands, feet, and side. Because of the presence of stigmatic marks, parts of her body were detached to be used as relics. There are eyewitness testimonies asserting that one such stigmatic mark was visible on St. Catherine's foot 217 years after her death. The foot is still intact and on display at the church of St. John and Paul in Venice. Many other saints have also been dismembered and the relics that have been distributed among various churches have also remained whole. This process of moving saintly relics from their original place of burial to a shrine is known as "translation."

A communal grave
St. Charbel Makhlouf died in 1898 at the Hermitage of St. Peter and St. Paul in Annaya, Lebanon. He was buried according to the strictures of his order, without a coffin and in a communal grave.

UNNATURAL INDICATIONS
Father Herbert Thurston (1856-1939), was a British priest, historian, and writer who specialized in parapsychology. While researching incorruptibility, he noted six key factors:
◆ An absence of rigor mortis.
◆ An absence of putrefaction.
◆ A pleasing fragrance given off by the incorrupted body.
◆ Bleeding from stigmata or wounds suffered in martyrdom.
◆ In rare cases, the conservation of body warmth over a long time.
◆ Even more rarely, the performing of a ritualized movement (such as the hand making the sign of the cross).

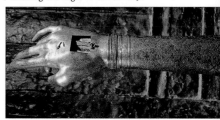

The act of "translation"
A hand and part of the skull of St. John the Baptist are said to be encased in these mountings.

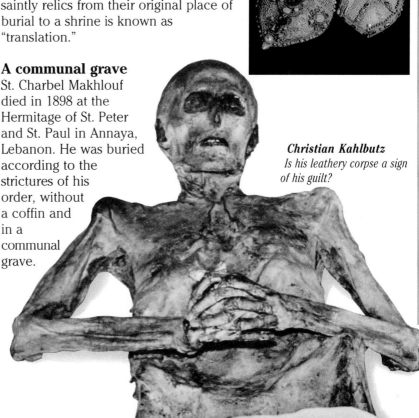

Christian Kahlbutz
Is his leathery corpse a sign of his guilt?

St. Charbel

The 19th-century monk St. Charbel Makhlouf is one of many saintly corpses surviving the ravages of time and moisture. His body was discovered intact floating in a muddy grave. Wet conditions usually speed putrefaction.

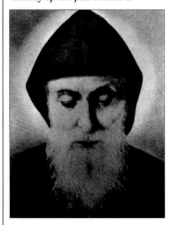

MUMMIFICATION

Some civilizations have tried to halt decomposition deliberately. Preservation of a corpse was an important part of ancient Egyptian religious belief. Influential citizens underwent the process called mummification. Internal organs were removed and the body immersed first in a solution of salt and then in natron, an embalming powder. After treatment with resin, the body was wrapped in oil-soaked bandages.

Defying decay

In fact, dead bodies can escape putrefaction through a varied combination of conditions that occur naturally. Moisture is the main agent encouraging decay. That is why hot, dry climates such as that found in Egypt have been very conducive to the preservation of bodies. Some sites are especially suitable and these have been identified and used as burial grounds by a number of civilizations throughout human history.

Corpses decayed normally all around him, and violent rainstorms sweeping the region turned the burial pit into a water-logged swamp. For 45 nights following his burial the devout monks of the monastery saw a bright light hovering in the air above the grave, which they interpreted as a sign of divine favor. After much prayer, the monastery superiors decided on an exhumation. When the saint's grave was opened four months after his death, his body was undecayed.

Miraculous fluid

After his exhumation, St. Charbel's body lay on display in the monastery's chapel for 29 years. During that time, an oily mixture of blood and perspiration seeped continually from the body. It became so profuse that the soiled clothing needed to be changed at least twice a week.

For 45 nights following St. Charbel's burial the devout monks of the monastery saw a bright light hovering in the air above the grave.

Pieces of the discarded robes (which were impregnated with the seemingly miraculous body fluid) were used as a healing agent for the incurably sick. In 1927 the body was medically examined by two physicians from the French Medical Institute in Beirut. Following the examination the saint's body was placed

Egyptian ruler

The head of the Egyptian pharaoh Rameses I was preserved by mummification. He lived well over 1,000 years before the birth of Christ.

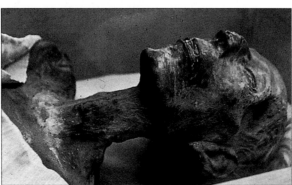

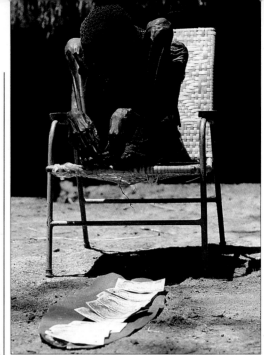

Deathly pose

A mummified body that was put on view to the public in Papua New Guinea.

in a new wooden coffin covered in zinc. The doctor's reports confirming the incorruptibility were sealed in a zinc tube, which was placed at the corpse's feet. The coffin was then bricked into a niche in the monastery wall. St. Charbel remained undisturbed until 1950, when pilgrims to the shrine noticed liquid oozing through a crevice in the wall. At another exhumation, ecclesiastical and medical authorities testified that St. Charbel's body was still lifelike, flexible, and free from any putrefaction. Every year since then, the tomb has been opened ceremoniously and the body is always in perfect condition. The liquid that has collected in the coffin is siphoned off and distributed among those seeking a miraculous cure.

Second skin

Saponification is a rare natural process by which body fats turn into a soap-like substance, thus preserving corpses in a lifelike state. The substance is known popularly as grave-wax, or *gras de cadavre* (French for "corpse fat"). Many corpses were discovered in a saponified condition during the clearance of the cemetery of the Church of Holy Innocents, now the Marché des Innocents, in Paris in 1785. The bodies showed no sign of decay. Even hair and eyes were completely whole five years or more after death and burial.

It is likely that saponification was responsible for some cases of alleged incorruption. Blessed Marie de Sainte-Euphrasie Pelletier died in 1868 and was

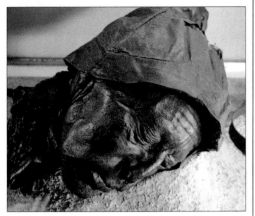

Human sacrifice
This sacrificial head was discovered in Denmark. Peat bogs are conducive to such preservation. Several perfectly intact bodies from the Iron Age have been found in Scotland, Ireland, and Denmark.

buried in a lead coffin. She was found to be still whole 35 years later, with even her eyelashes intact. One of the doctors present wrote: "...we were able to ascertain that the chest, the abdomen, the thighs and the legs were covered with a skin like that of a mummy, under which was a mass of *gras de cadavre*, resulting from the saponification of the tissues which remained underneath."

A second doctor noted that the skin was "mummy-like, hard to the touch, and resonant when struck by any kind of metal instrument...."

Twelve years had passed but the baby's body was found to be entirely intact.

Authenticated cases of what seems like true incorruption are rare, but they do exist. A modern example concerned Nadia Mattei who died in Rome in 1965, aged two. Soon after the funeral, her distraught mother had dreams in which the dead child appeared to be begging to be fetched from the grave. The dreams persisted and Signora Mattei began petitioning for an exhumation. At first the authorities treated her as just a poor mother demented with grief. But her persistence won out. Finally, in early 1977 her request was granted. Twelve years had passed, but baby Nadia's body was found to be entirely intact when the coffin was opened. The case defied any rational explanation and was reported in newspapers all around the world.

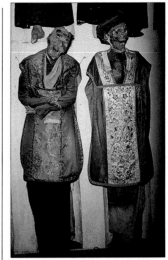

Sicilian cemetery
If the conditions are right, some bodies are preserved naturally.

Lasting conditions
These "natural" mummies were found in the crypt of a church in Sàvoca, Sicily. Some bodies have survived over 250 years in Sicilian catacombs without being reduced to skeletons.

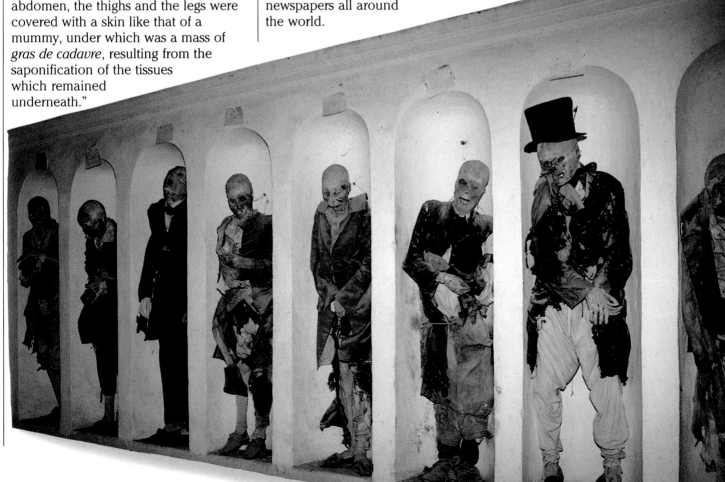

Indian fakirs are famous for their ascetic practices. They believe that mortification of the flesh is the road to spiritual enlightenment. While some keep constantly on the move, others stay motionless until their limbs atrophy. Their bodies may become homes for insects or birds.

Bed of nails
Discipline and discomfort are used to reach a holy state.

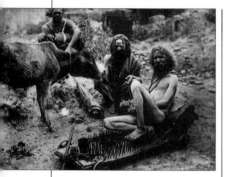

Some fakirs keep their fists clenched so that their fingernails grow into the flesh of their palms. Others hold their faces upturned until the neck muscles freeze and the position becomes permanent. Fakirs may lie for long periods on beds of nails or even remain in water for weeks at a time.

Skin and bones
Fakirs believe that the endurance of physical hardship helps their spiritual concentration.

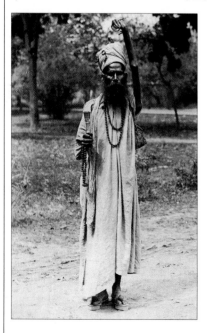

SUSPENDING LIFE

Holy men, yogis, and fakirs use religious faith to help them take control of their own bodies. Some appear able to survive for a long time without water, air, or food. How do they achieve this mysterious ability to cheat death?

INCORRUPTIBLES ARE DEAD HUMANS who seem to defy the usual rules of decomposition. There are other people, just as remarkable, who allow themselves to be buried alive – and are found alive days and even months later.

A classic story involves an Indian yogi called Haridas who became famous for being buried alive for a period of four months. News of this reached the maharaja of Lahore, who skeptically asked for a repetition of the feat under controlled conditions.

Harrowing preparations
The *Calcutta Medical Times* told the story of Haridas's preparations in 1835. Apparently he cut away muscles under his tongue so that it could be folded back to close nasal passages at the back of the throat. The yogi ate only milk and yoghurt for days before his burial, and he bathed in hot water. Then he swallowed a long strip of linen and regurgitated it to clean his alimentary canal, before embarking on a total fast. Haridas closed his nose and ears with wax and settled into a cross-legged pose. Doctors found that his pulse had virtually stopped.

Unearthing the yogi
Haridas was then wrapped in linen, put in a padlocked chest and buried; barley was sown in the ground above the chest. A wall was built around the site and guards were posted. A full 40 days later an expectant crowd gathered to see the chest opened. The barley on the ground above had grown undisturbed. Locks on the chest were untouched. The shrouded yogi was found inside, in exactly the same pose.

As an eyewitness, British general Sir Claude Wade reported on the yogi's condition. Haridas had no detectable pulse, his arms and legs had shrunk and were stiff. But doctors massaged Haridas, pulled back his tongue, emptied his ears of wax and inflated his lungs with bellows. Eventually signs of life appeared. Within a few hours, Haridas was fully restored to the land of the living. The doubting maharaja rewarded him with diamonds.

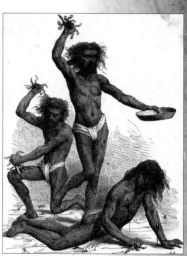

Inflicting pain
Yogic practices may seem strange – but they show that we are all capable of great self-control.

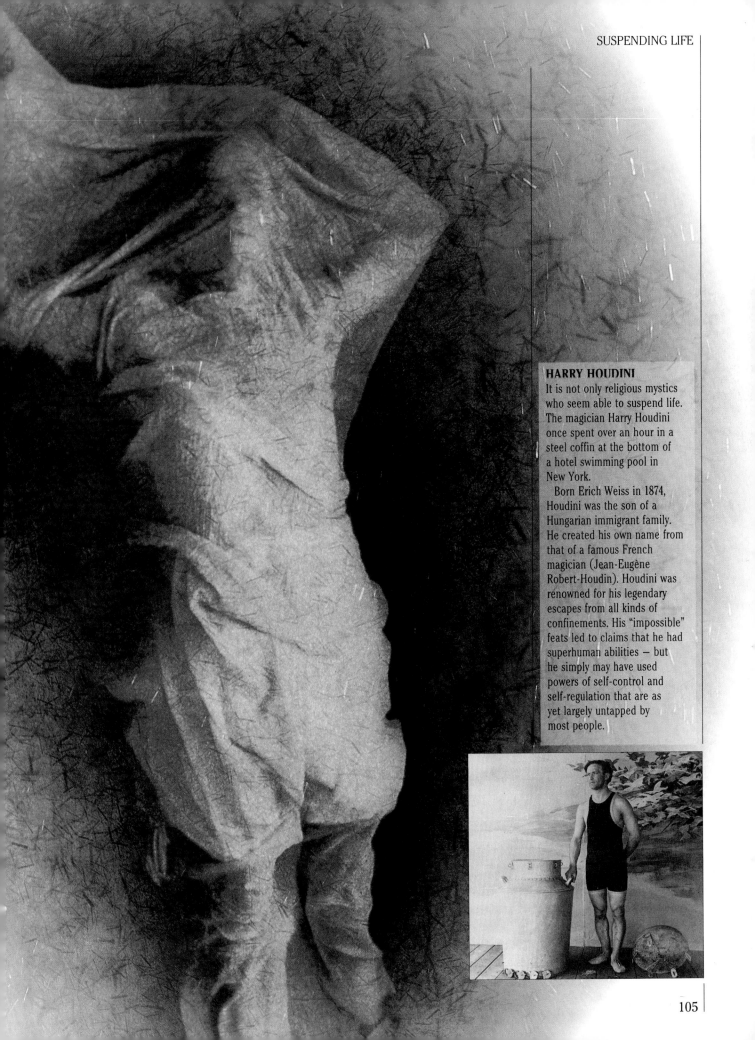

HARRY HOUDINI

It is not only religious mystics who seem able to suspend life. The magician Harry Houdini once spent over an hour in a steel coffin at the bottom of a hotel swimming pool in New York.

Born Erich Weiss in 1874, Houdini was the son of a Hungarian immigrant family. He created his own name from that of a famous French magician (Jean-Eugène Robert-Houdin). Houdini was renowned for his legendary escapes from all kinds of confinements. His "impossible" feats led to claims that he had superhuman abilities — but he simply may have used powers of self-control and self-regulation that are as yet largely untapped by most people.

RASPUTIN

Grigori Rasputin, a self-styled holy man, born in 1871, was notorious both for his debauchery and for the influence he exercised over the Russian royal family. He was also reputed to be a healer and a man of strange mystical powers. When assassins confronted him in 1916, he proved nearly impossible to kill. First, they served him poisoned cakes and wine – but these had no effect. Then he was shot and left for dead in a locked room.

Grigori Rasputin

Unnatural strength

Less than an hour later, Rasputin burst open the locked door and escaped. He was in full flight when two further shots hit him. His assassins tied his hands, bundled his unconscious body into a waiting car, and drove to the frozen river Neva, where they dumped his body through the broken ice. Rasputin's daughter Maria reported that when his corpse was found, his right hand was frozen to his chest. She said it was as though he were making the Christian sign of the cross.

Buried alive

Egyptian Rahman Bey's live burial in Carshalton, Surrey, England, in 1938 is shown here. When dug up hours later, he was found to be in good condition.

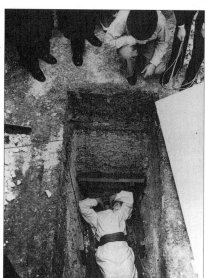

Yogis in India have accomplished extraordinary feats that appear to transcend physical laws. They practice a Hindu system of philosophy that aims at a mystical union of self with a Supreme Being. A daily routine of mental and physical exercises enables yogis to take almost complete control of their bodies. As a result, they are able to survive situations that would normally lead to terrible injuries or death. Yogis may try also to suspend

Careful balance
This Sri Lankan yogi appears to be held up by only a strong will and a very thin stick.

breathing for astonishingly long periods. They may show different pulse rates on each wrist and survive in a trance state for weeks without any food or water. The persistent effort necessary to sustain years of self-discipline apparently gives Yogis conscious control over the autonomic nervous system that governs the body's involuntary functions. A skilled yogi aims to control not only pulse rate and breathing but also such functions as body temperature and kidney activity. Live burial is the ultimate demonstration of the power of the mind over the body. A yogi does not lose consciousness during such a burial but is rather in a state of

very deep and controlled meditation. Stories abound about the incredible feats achieved by Indian holy men. Some are said to have survived long periods with their heads buried in the earth. Others have been buried with their arms held above their heads for more than 30 years.

Many tales may be exaggerated but there seem to be credible witnesses to at least some of these unusual feats. Simulated deaths have been witnessed elsewhere as well. For example, a legendary story from Africa concerns an entire village in what was the British Cameroons, now known as Cameroon, in 1932. A sergeant in the Native Bush Police was sent to a village in the Ibibio tribal territory to find out why the villagers were refusing to pay their taxes. At first he thought the village was deserted, until he discovered the entire population hiding from him by sitting in open-work baskets in eight feet of water. They appeared to be asleep, with their vital functions suspended. The sergeant was unable to wake them, and had to leave without the taxes.

In 1950 *The Lancet* (a respected British medical journal) reported the following yogic feat. A yogi by the name of Shri Ramdasji was put into a cubicle and buried. After 56 hours a hole was bored into the box lid, 1,400 gallons of water poured in, and the hole re-sealed. Seven hours later the yogi was found submerged – but still quite alive.

Punishing the flesh to purify the spirit is an ancient practice. The ascetics of the Syrian and Egyptian deserts of the fourth and fifth centuries A.D. were renowned for the severity of their self discipline. One of them

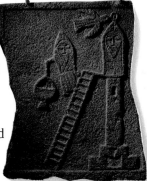

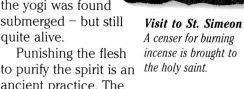

Visit to St. Simeon
A censer for burning incense is brought to the holy saint.

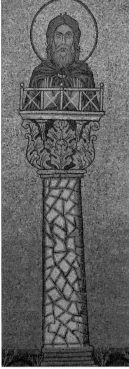

Column dweller
St. Simeon is depicted on his pillar in this mosaic.

burdened his body with so many chains that he had to crawl around like an animal. Another lived on a diet of seeds, while yet another spent most of his life at the bottom of a dried-up well. Most celebrated was Simeon Stylites, a fifth-century Christian saint. As a young monk he lived in Tellneshin, near Antioch in Syria (now Antakya in Turkey). He persuaded a local abbot to wall him up in his cell for the 40 days of Lent with just 10 loaves of bread and a jug of water. After 40 days, Simeon was found unconscious, with the bread and water untouched. He went on to observe a total fast during Lent for the rest of his life.

Simeon lived until the age of 70, and spent 42 of those years perched on a tiny platform atop a 60-foot pillar in the Arabian desert. He endured both the sun by day and the bitter cold by night. Simeon preached several sermons a day and prayed all night with his arms raised high to heaven. After he died, a great church was constructed at Qalaat Semaan. This church was unique in that its main focus was Simeon's pillar and not the usual altar. Many ascetics were inspired to follow his example. These people became known as Stylites.

It appears that the bodily control needed for feats of suspended animation

Cloister ruins
Syrian ruins of the Simeon cloisters are a reminder of the saintly ascetic.

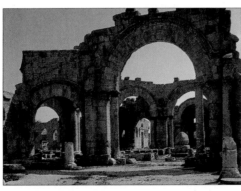

Simeon spent 42 years perched on a tiny platform atop a 60-foot pillar.

may be acquired through practice. But some people seem to have an innate talent to withstand difficult conditions that most people would find unbearable.

One example is the case of Nathan Coker, whose ability to withstand intense heat was reported in the *New York Herald* in 1871. Coker was neither a showman nor a religious fanatic, but a blacksmith. He had always just accepted his "gift" as a rather useful fact of life. As he became a celebrity in his hometown of Easton, Maryland, the local citizens demanded a demonstration. Coker began by heating a shovel in his forge until it was white hot. He then removed his heavy boots and pressed the searing metal against the soles of his bare feet. Next, he heated lead and swilled the molten metal around in his mouth. When he spat it out, the lead had solidified.

As his stunned audience gaped in amazement, Coker thrust his hands into the furnace, leisurely selected several glowing coals and paraded them around on his palms. He ended his display by picking up a piece of red-hot iron from the blazing hearth and turning it over in his hands. He had no burns and was unharmed.

The existence of "ordinary" people who have "superhuman" abilities suggests that people may have more potential to control their bodies than they realize. The yogis in India who are buried alive may point to a higher potential in us all. Most people are not concerned with performing amazing tricks — but the abilities could have a real benefit in helping to fight disease.

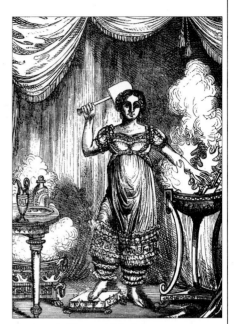

Fireproof lady?
Madame Giraldelli was a famous performer at 19th-century English fairs. Her act included placing melted lead in her mouth, thrusting her arm into fire, and washing her hands in boiling oil.

Body states
Being buried alive may seem like hibernation, but the processes are quite different. In hibernation, the metabolic rate (the energy required to keep the body functioning at rest) is lowered and the blood sugar supply is reduced. But although the pulse rate drops during the trance induced prior to live burial, the metabolic rate is high and blood sugar supply remains the same or may even rise.

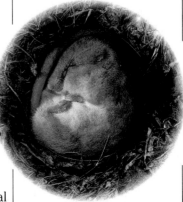

A hibernating dormouse

AN ACT OF WILL

"Humankind has more talents and more potential for self-regulation than we...use or take credit for."
Elmer and Alyce Green, *Beyond Biofeedback*

EOPLE DON'T USUALLY consciously decide to breathe, or instruct their hearts to beat. Fortunately, some of our body processes are involuntary and normally keep happening without us having to think about them. What is impressive about yogis and others who manage amazing feats of endurance is that they seem to be able to exercise conscious control over some of these processes.

Feeding back information

But recent research shows that ordinary people can learn such skills. Biofeedback training techniques are tools for helping people to regulate involuntary body functions. Most of these techniques were pioneered in the 1950's and 1960's. The feedback they provide is simply information on the activity levels of involuntary processes – such as blood pressure, heart rate, and acid secretion in the digestive system. Patients use this feedback to monitor their ability to control these various body activities.

For example, patients can receive feedback in the form of colored lights. Research projects in the 1970's used three lights. A green light told the patient to try to speed up the heart, a red light was the signal to slow down the heart, and a yellow light stayed on whenever the heart rate was right. All the patients learned to control their heart rate to some degree. Many doctors now accept that such training may help in treating conditions such as anxiety, hypertension (high blood pressure), and migraine. Researchers are now starting to apply the techniques to other problems and disorders, such as AIDS.

During biofeedback training, the mind focuses on the desired effect. This is not in itself a therapy and does not have any inherent power to cure. However, it can contribute, along with relaxation and meditation techniques, to the efficiency of the body's own innate

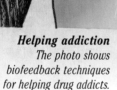

Helping addiction
The photo shows biofeedback techniques for helping drug addicts.

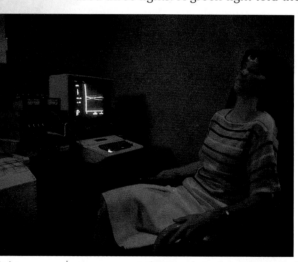

BIOFEEDBACK TRAINING

Biofeedback training was developed in the U.S. in the 1960's. The training aims to teach the patient to control his or her unconscious body activities, including blood pressure, pulse rate, body temperature, muscle tension, the amount of sweat on the skin, brain waves, and stomach acidity. First, a doctor links the patient to a recording instrument that measures the relevant process. The instrument provides some signal, such as a flashing light, a fluctuating needle on a meter, or a changing sound tone, so that the patient can monitor how well he or she is controlling activity.

For example, a man with high blood pressure is linked to a biofeedback machine and then tries to lower his pressure reading. As he succeeds, a light starts to flash. He becomes aware of how he feels when the light flashes. By responding to the light, he gradually acquires the ability to lower blood pressure at will. Eventually, the patient has such firm control that he can lower his blood pressure at any time, without the help of a biofeedback machine.

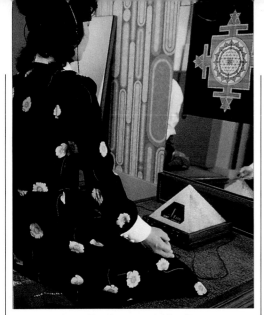

A meditation center in Japan
The pyramid-shaped indicator shows how deeply a subject is meditating. The color red indicates "asleep," and green suggests "concentration."

healing system. Biofeedback is regarded by many people as especially useful when used to alleviate disorders that are aggravated by stress or tension.

In 1967 an American pyschologist, Neal Miller, reported on biofeedback experiments with rats. In laboratory boxes, Miller's rats were rewarded by having the pleasure center of their brains stimulated. This kind of positive reward encouraged the rats to respond to signals in a certain way. The rats actually learned to raise or lower their blood pressure and control their heart rates. Further experiments showed that rats could control their kidneys as well.

Brain wave training
Also in the 1960's, the Chicago-based neuropsychiatrist Joe Kamiya independently investigated the relationship between physical states and brain wave activity. Every time a bell sounded students were asked to guess what brain wave they were producing. The students quickly learned to identify waves correctly. Eventually they were able to switch at will from one brain wave to another. Such training was tried with epileptics in the 1970's. Some patients were able to produce desired brain waves and reduce the frequency of epileptic fits.

The roots of today's biofeedback theories lie in earlier techniques of auto-suggestion. Practitioners of these techniques did not use machines, but rather trained their subjects to become more aware of their bodies' involuntary functions. Dr. Johannes Schulz published his book on autogenic training in 1932. The exercises he pioneered have helped people with various disorders. For example, asthma sufferers have been able to learn to control the rhythm of their breathing using this technique.

Self-healing
Elmer and Alyce Green of the Menninger Foundation in Topeka, Kansas, devised a new therapeutic method that combined elements of both Schulz's autogenic training and Kamiya's technique. Great emphasis was placed on visualization as a powerful instrument of self-healing. In their 1977 book *Beyond Biofeedback*, the Greens described how 150 terminally ill cancer patients with less than a year to live were taught to envisage diseased cells of the body being dispersed and

> # "It's as if your body has always been on automatic pilot, and suddenly you find you can take over the controls."
> ### Laboratory volunteer

destroyed. Using self-hypnosis, each patient was encouraged to create his or her own individual fantasy. A keen chess player might "see" cancer cells as pawns being beaten off the board. Another person might see the cells as small fish being swallowed by an attacking shark.

The results were very encouraging: 22 percent of the cancers regressed completely, 19 percent showed evidence of remission, and 27 percent stabilized. The remaining 32 percent of patients did die, but it was estimated that they had prolonged their lives by about a year.

Many in the medical profession accept that the mind can exercise some control over the autonomic nervous system. While there are doubts as to how much control is possible, many patients are being encouraged to at least try a more active role in restoring their own health. Biofeedback techniques are an important way of establishing this patient power.

MAN OF FREE WILL
One of the earliest practitioners of self-healing by auto-suggestion was the 19th-century philosopher and psychologist William James.

As a young medical student James fell ill while on a trip to the Amazon. He became interested in the idea of free will and how a person could use thought to affect the body. He consciously attempted to influence his health by positive thought and noticed that this produced a marked improvement in his condition.

In 1872 James was appointed to teach physiology at Harvard, where he subsequently taught psychology as a laboratory science. In 1890 James published *The Principles of Psychology*, which contained an exposition of his philosophy of free will and the power of the mind to influence the body.

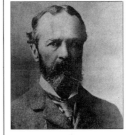

William James

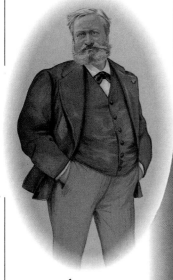

Émile Zola

Ancient Rome
This relief decoration comes from a Roman tomb. To prevent a premature diagnosis of death, the Romans did not perform funerary rites until eight days after death.

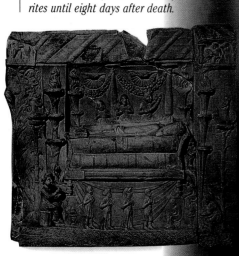

FATAL ASSUMPTIONS

Before the days of sophisticated medical knowledge and modern diagnostic tools, people who fell into a coma or were paralyzed were sometimes mistakenly left for dead — and even buried alive!

IN MARCH 1990, an American who had been in a coma for 10 years was given the tranquilizer Valium in preparation for dental work. Within minutes he was awake and starting to talk. To the astonishment of his neurologist, Dr. A. Kanner, the man knew not only his name, the names of his family and where he used to work, but could perform extremely complicated mental arithmetic as well.

Although this patient had been in a coma from which he was not expected to recover, his family and physicians were all aware that he was "technically" still alive. There have been many instances, particularly in the early days of medical science, where the misleading appearance of death has led to a very premature burial.

Her eyes could move up or down on command, but she could close her left eyelid only partially. Her jaw was clenched tightly and there was a total paralysis of the tongue, palate, pharynx, and neck.

Bernard le Bovier de Fontanelle, an 18th-century French scientific philosopher, recorded 46 cases of living people who were mistakenly buried as dead. In order to prevent this, the ancient Greeks had passed a law stipulating that no "dead" person should be buried until six or seven days after the pronouncement of death. For the same reason, the ancient Romans waited until the eighth day before they performed last rites.

Mistaken for dead

One of the medical conditions that might have led to a mistaken verdict of death is catalepsy. This is a state in which the muscles of the face, body, and limbs are stuck in a semi-rigid position. Neither the body posture nor facial expression alters, sometimes for many hours. Catalepsy occurs primarily in people with schizophrenia, epilepsy, or a conversion disorder (in which painful emotions are repressed by unconsciously converting them into some kind of physical symptoms).

Another condition that may have been mistaken for death is "locked-in" syndrome. This is usually caused by a brain hemorrhage or blood clot, and results in a state of almost total paralysis. The sufferer is rendered mute and unable to move any muscles except for those controlling the eyeballs and eyelids, but remains fully conscious throughout the experience. Unless someone is alert enough to notice eye movement, the diagnosis will be profound coma. The following case was one of seven dealing with this this fairly rare affliction in the *British Medical Journal*, November 1974.

No way out

In February 1973 a seemingly healthy 35-year-old housewife developed neck pain, followed immediately by dizziness, double vision and very slurred speech. Within 24 hours, she was unable to move any limbs or muscles except for those of the eye and eyelid. Her eyes could move up or down on command, but she could close her left eyelid only partially. Her jaw was clenched tightly and there was a total paralysis of the tongue, palate, pharynx, and neck. Helplessly trapped inside her own body,

she was mercifully released when she died of a respiratory infection six weeks later. Other people may be condemned to suffer their conscious hell for as long as a year. Recognition of the locked-in state is extremely important, not least because the patient's hearing is perfectly intact. One can imagine the anguish that could be suffered when, thinking the person is in a mindless coma, doctors and family discuss sensitive issues.

She suffered an entire hour of intense pain under the surgeon's knife before she finally managed to move a finger.

A similar – if temporary – state of locked-in helplessness is experienced by those who wake during an operation to find themselves totally paralyzed by muscle-relaxing drugs and unable to signal that they are not properly anesthetized.

In March 1990, 44-year-old Pamela Hill was awarded £55,000 (about $90,000) damages by a British crown court for the torture she endured as she lay awake during a hysterectomy. As reported in the *Guardian* newspaper on March 16, 1990, she suffered an entire hour of intense pain before she managed to move a finger and alert the anesthetist. High damages were also awarded to another Englishwoman, from the county of Shropshire. She woke at the first cut of the knife when her baby was being delivered by Cesarean section. She eventually managed to wiggle a toe but unfortunately no one present noticed her helpless plight.

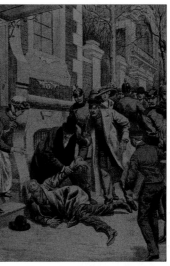

Dropping in the street
The sleeping sickness epidemic claims another victim, this time in the streets of Berlin.

SLEEPING SICKNESS
(Encephalitis lethargica)
There are few survivors of the great sleeping sickness epidemic that occurred earlier this century, but their story is an extraordinary example of the "living dead" awakening. After starting in Vienna in 1916, the virus raged for 10 years, spreading across Europe and to North America, and affecting some five million people. (It is likely that the even more widespread influenza pandemic that happened at the same time lowered resistance to sleeping sickness.) Virus-borne encephalitis lethargica is different from the African sleeping sickness (trypanosomiasis) which is parasite-borne.

Lack of energy
Many victims died and survivors often failed to recover their liveliness. They would sit motionless, speechless, and without any energy or motivation to act.

Hundreds of thousands of these patients died in nursing homes or other institutions, largely forgotten by society. Yet some people managed to live on in their isolated, half-conscious state.

Forgotten victims
When Dr. Oliver Sacks, the eminent British neurologist, arrived at Mount Carmel Hospital in New York in 1966, he encountered 80 of these post-encephalitic patients, one of the few such groups left in the world. Nearly half were virtually speechless and could hardly move. In 1969 a new drug called L-dopa was tried on some of these patients and produced amazing results. In his book *Awakenings* Dr. Sacks described the effect the drug had on a female patient: "She surfaced and shot into the air like a cork released." She soon began talking very excitedly: "I'm a brand-new person" she said. "It is so long since I had any feelings...."

THE LIVING DEAD

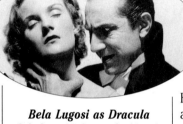

Bela Lugosi as Dracula
Bela Lugosi is known for his role as Dracula in the 1931 film. The actor grew so attached to the part that he asked to be buried in the cloak he wore for the role.

Buried alive

People have been mistakenly buried alive more often than is generally acknowledged. Various devices have been invented to enable victims to summon help. One apparatus included a tube and a ball that lay on the chest of the deceased. Any movement from the body moved the ball, resulting in a signal at ground level. The signal indicated that a door in the coffin should be opened to let in light and air.

In early 19th-century New York the chances of being buried alive were as high as one in every 200 bodies. A new ordinance at that time required coffins ready for burial to be kept above ground for eight days, and open at the head. Strings attached to bells were tied to the "corpse's" hands and feet, so that the slightest movement of the bodies would ring the bells. Out of 1,200 bodies so arranged, six bodies "returned to life."

"A Vampyr is a dead body which continues to live in the grave; which it leaves, however, by night, for the purpose of sucking the blood of the living, whereby it is nourished and preserved in good condition, instead of becoming decomposed like other dead bodies."
Georg Conrad Horst, 1821

THE VAMPIRE IS A REPULSIVE but thoroughly compelling supernatural creature. Early examples of vampirism can be found in the blood-sucking demons and spirits of ancient mythology. But belief in such creatures has been especially strong in eastern and central Europe, and the vampire emerged from 16th-century Balkan states in the form we would recognize today. By the 17th century, travelers returning from those parts brought spine-chilling tales of blood-sucking and possession. A vampire "panic" in 18th-century Hungary was so widespread that it was investigated by a royal commission. The image of the vampire also stimulated the creative imagination of various 19th-century writers. Goethe, Byron, and Baudelaire all wrote vampire-inspired verses. Vampire plays were staged all over Europe, vampire cabaret acts were performed, and in Germany there was even a production of a vampire opera.

Bram Stoker's Dracula

It was the 1897 publication of Bram Stoker's *Dracula*, a Gothic tale of gore and horror, that established the enduring notoriety of the vampire Count Dracula. Stoker had based Count Dracula on a notorious 15th-century sadist, the feared and hated Romanian prince Vlad Tepes. As a result of his sadistic cruelty toward his enemies, many of whom suffered terrible deaths on his instruction, Tepes earned the alternative title of Vlad the Impaler. His nickname "Drakula" is actually the Romanian word meaning "son of the devil."

Magical powers

The enduring myth is that a vampire is a corpse that returns to a lifelike state and sucks human blood. Witches, demons, and other malevolent spirits are motivated by an evil desire for revenge or the corruption of innocence. But a vampire is driven by its endless thirst for fresh blood. For a vampire, the

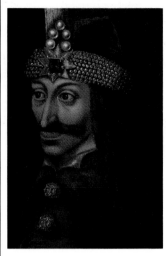

"Son of the devil"
Vlad Tepes was a 15th-century sadist who became the real-life model for Bram Stoker's fictional Count Dracula.

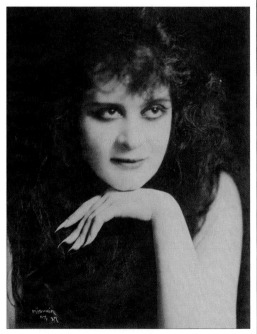

Screen vamp
The image of the vampire is even found in Hollywood. Actress Theda Bara was the first of a generation of Hollywood vamps. The character she portrayed on screen devoured her male victims in a figurative way. The title vamp derived from Bara's full red lips and dark, fascinating eyes — similar to those of a vampire.

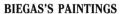

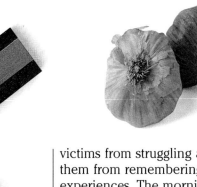

Antivampire devices
Garlic, salt, and the crucifix are thought to drive vampires away.

Despite its awesome supernatural powers a vampire is not totally invulnerable.

sucking of blood is a form of transfusion — a way of trying to restore its life and resist decomposition. Folklore has endowed this ghoulish creature with many supernatural powers. It can climb in and out of a grave through six feet of hard-packed earth. It can take on such forms as a wolf or a bat — then change as easily into a cloud of mist. In this way, a vampire may seep through keyholes and under doors.

Hypnotic powers
Vampires also have a mysterious power over animals. Legends tell of wolves, cats, owls, rats, and even flies that have been charmed into aiding heinous activities. The vampire is also a capable hypnotist. It uses this talent to stop victims from struggling and to prevent them from remembering their terrifying experiences. The morning after a vampire attack, victims know only a strange tiredness, which they think is a result of the bizarre nightmares that have disturbed their sleep.

According to popular belief, anyone receiving a vampire's bite will then become a vampire. Other potential vampires have included people who have committed suicide, died under a curse, or been buried without proper rites. Anyone thought different or in any way unusual could come under suspicion. Harelips, blue eyes, red hair, odd birthmarks, and babies born with teeth have all been interpreted as signs of the vampire. A universally accepted image today is of a gaunt, pale creature with long, sharp teeth, fleshy lips, particularly bad breath, and cruel, mesmerizing eyes.

Despite its awesome supernatural powers a vampire is not totally invulnerable. It can function only at night and lies helpless in its grave or tomb during the day. A vampire cannot cross water, is kept at bay by garlic, and actively fears the crucifix in any form.

Once it is cornered, the vampire can be destroyed with a silver bullet (ideally made from a melted-down crucifix), or

Japanese vampire
The Vampire Cat of Nabeshima is an example from the Far East of the vampire myth. The story goes that the huge cat killed a prince's favorite concubine, assumed her form, and tormented the unfortunate prince.

BIEGAS'S PAINTINGS
The fantastic vampires painted by Polish artist Boleslas Biegas appear very sensual. The activities of vampires, particularly those on screen, do have strong sexual overtones. Dracula's victim is usually a beautiful young woman. The drawing of blood often takes place in a bedroom.

A vampire first caresses its victim with soothing, stroking movements before plunging unnaturally long, razor-sharp canine teeth into the victim's neck.

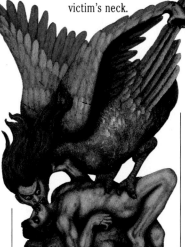

"Kiss of Vampire," 1916
A painting by Boleslas Biegas.

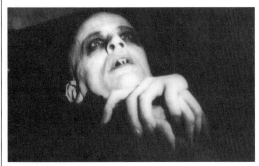

Nosferatu
Actor Klaus Kinski continued the vampire tradition in the 1979 movie, Nosferatu, the Vampyre, *directed by Werner Herzog.*

While such a creature seems pure fantasy, there is a real but rare medical condition called Congenital Erythropoietic Porphyria that may have encouraged the idea. This condition results in excessive hair growth on the face, arms, and legs. Both teeth and urine are colored red. A sufferer becomes very pale and should not venture out into sunlight, as this causes severe skin blistering.

Vampire bat
Like the legendary vampire, the common vampire bat feeds on blood, drawn mainly from livestock. Native to Mexico and South America, the bat does not suck the blood of its victims, but laps it up with its tongue after piercing the skin with its teeth. The vampire bat is a small reddish-brown mammal about three inches long. It has razor-sharp, triangular-shaped incisors, and an esophagus that allows only fluids to pass. People fear the bat's bite primarily because it has been known to carry rabies.

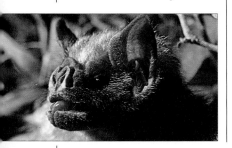

by having a stake driven through the heart. Traditionally, the stake must be cut from hawthorn or aspen wood. According to some conventions, only one blow can be used to drive this stake home. (The old British custom of piercing the bodies of suicides with a stake was rooted in the fear of vampires. This practice survived until it was forbidden by law in 1824.)

Real-life vampire personalities with a thirst for blood have existed. The first recorded case was that of Gilles de Rais, a sadistic 15th-century French baron. Although showing courage when fighting alongside Joan of Arc, it was his cruelty and perversions that earned him infamy. He and his associates indulged in horrific orgies, which often included disemboweling live children and drinking their blood. Known appropriately as the Black Baron, he was finally executed for his crimes in 1440.

> **The countess kept many terrified young girls chained in her dark dungeons to be "milked" whenever she was taken by a blood-thirst.**

Another infamous blood-lusting monster was the Hungarian noblewoman Countess Elisabeth Bathory. She was born in 1560 to a life of luxury. Her hideous deviation first showed when she struck out during a temper tantrum and gashed her maid with a comb. Some blood splashed onto her hands and she was seized by a sudden, strange, and compelling urge to lick it. Despite widespread rumors, it was many years before the authorities raided her castle. What they found was worse than anyone could have imagined. The countess not only drank blood but bathed in it as well. She kept many

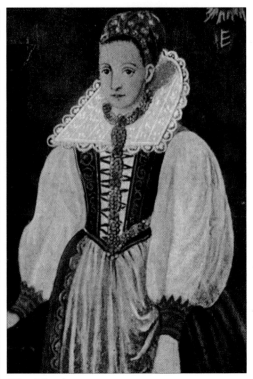

Blood-lusting monster
In the 16th century Hungarian Countess Elisabeth Bathory murdered young girls and drank their blood.

terrified young girls chained in her dark dungeons to be "milked" whenever she was taken by a blood-thirst. By the time she was brought to trial in 1611, the countess was said to have murdered hundreds of young girls for their blood. Her accomplices were all beheaded, but Elisabeth Bathory's fate was more protracted. She was walled-up in her own bedroom and left to die a slow, painful death.

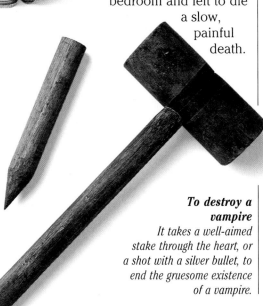

To destroy a vampire
It takes a well-aimed stake through the heart, or a shot with a silver bullet, to end the gruesome existence of a vampire.

ZOMBIES — THE WALKING DEAD

A zombie is a soulless corpse that is raised from the grave and given a half-life by a sorcerer with voodoo powers. Without any willpower or intelligence, the dazed creature blindly obeys the sorcerer's every wicked command.

VOODOO IS A RELIGIOUS CULT involving magical rites and trance-invoked communication with ancestral spirits. Voodoo beliefs originated in Africa and were then carried to the Caribbean by African slaves. In Haiti, where the voodoo tradition is strong, many people still delight in their supernatural folklore, and tales of zombies are related with considerable relish.

Practitioners of voodoo attempt to sell souls to the devil in return for favors. To obtain a soul a voodoo sorcerer, known as a *houngan*, goes to a victim's house, sucks out their soul, and traps it in a corked bottle. Without a soul, the victim soon falls ill and dies.

In order to turn the corpse into a zombie the sorcerer must return to the body as quickly as possible, while it is still fresh. At midnight on the burial day, the sorcerer opens the grave, calls the victim's name, and passes the bottle containing the soul under the corpse's nose.

Going to the grave

Families keep watch over new graves to prevent sorcerers from opening them. A body is often placed face-down in its grave with its mouth full of earth, so that it cannot answer if the sorcerer summons it. Sometimes heavy stone slabs are placed on graves to deter the sorcerers. But if a sorcerer reaches the corpse in time, the dead person becomes reanimated and is led from its place of rest as a zombie. The sorcerer then has a new soul to sell and a zombie slave to do his bidding.

According to popular legend, zombies are also used for the purpose of fortune-telling. To this end sorcerers perform dark rituals in remote

Zombie on show
A man wrapped in a shroud and with his face whitened takes part in a Haitian street festival. He is meant to represent a zombie.

African voodoo
Voodoo ceremonies like this one in Togo, West Africa, were the origin of rituals still performed in Haiti today.

cemeteries. They erect a crude wooden cross at the foot of a grave. The cross is draped with a frock coat and crowned by a silk top hat to create an effigy of the god of the dead, Baron Samedi. Three lighted candles are then placed at the foot of the cross and the effigy is showered with acacia, balsam, and assorted herbs while a sorcerer intones, "Dormi pa'fume, Baron Samedi" (sleep sweetly, Baron Samedi). The chosen body is then dug up and interrogated as to the location of a hidden stash of money or questioned regarding the future.

Zombies can only be released if given salt, either dissolved in water or mixed with food. Consumption of this "magic" ingredient allows a zombie to escape its tormented state of "living death" and eventually to return to the peace of its grave.

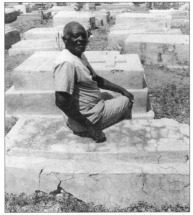

Graveside visit
Narcisse, a Haitian, claims that he died in May 1962, but was resurrected as a zombie. Here he sits proudly on what was his tomb.

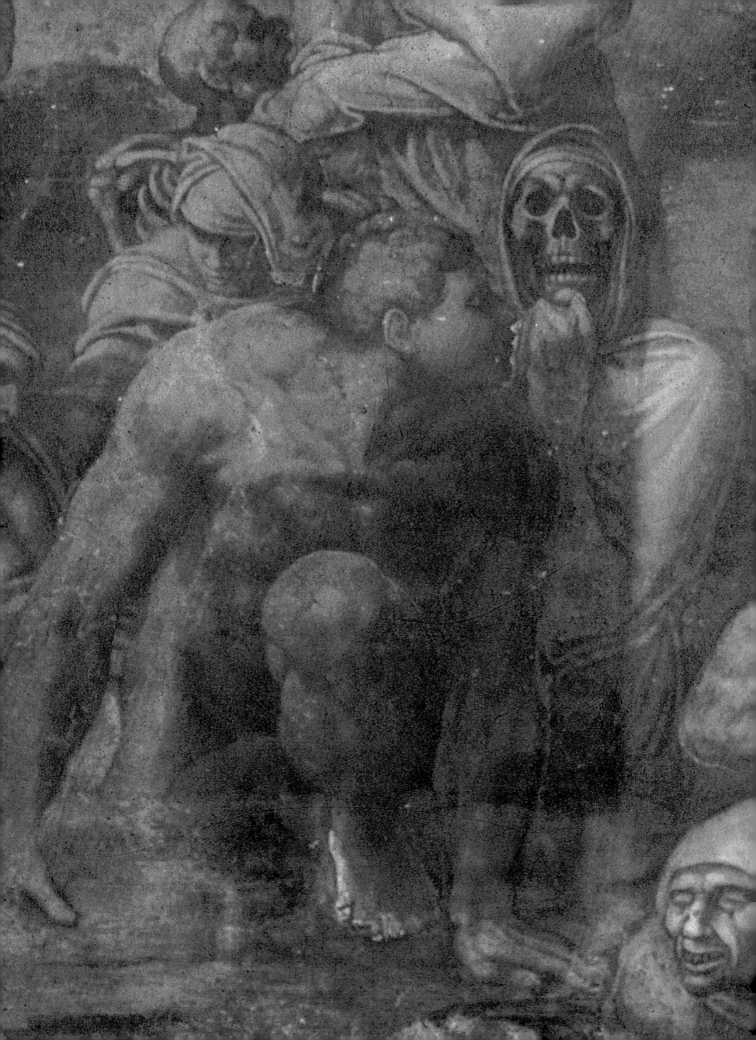

CHAPTER FIVE

AFTER THE JUDGMENT

Belief in life after death has been almost universal since early times. It is only in the last 150 years that the idea has been questioned by any sizable part of humankind. But reports from spiritualists who claim to see and hear the dead have served to reinforce ancient beliefs.

By studying the burial practices of early cultures it is possible to learn much about ancient attitudes to life after death. As long as 60,000 years ago, Neanderthal tribespeople disposed of their dead ceremoniously. In the later Stone Age, about 40,000 years ago, both graves and their contents became more elaborate.

For many cultures the method of burial, the preparation of the corpse, and the inclusion of specific objects in the grave were vital for a soul's continued existence. Numerous societies believed that a proper burial guaranteed a clear passage to the afterlife. But different peoples have their own opinions as to what constitutes a "proper" burial. Burial under the earth is only one method of disposing of the dead. Some cultures prefer to place bodies in caves or mounds above ground level. Other societies put corpses high above the earth, either in trees or on scaffolds. Burial at sea is common among seafaring communities.

Preservation

Many of the varied methods of burial reflect the widely held view that the body must be preserved, both from the rigors of climate and the attentions of animals seeking food, if its owner is to survive in the afterlife. Egyptians believed that the preservation of a corpse by way of mummification ensured a smooth transition into the next world. Initially this privilege was restricted to the Egyptian nobility, but gradually the burial rites of kings were made available to the aristocracy and then to anyone who could afford to pay for the careful, and expensive, process of mummification.

Wealthy Egyptians understood existence in the afterlife to be a purely pleasurable version of their earthly lives, and servants or models of servants were placed in tombs so that they could continue to serve their masters beyond the grave. Everyday goods, including

food and drink, were often buried with the dead for use in an afterlife. The Phoenicians built clay pipes running down from ground level to receptacles in burial chambers below. Wine was poured through these pipes to the dead, who had access to the receptacles through windows in their burial vaults.

Symbolic objects were also buried with corpses. For example, in ancient Mexico, small clay female figures were put in graves to ensure rebirth in a life after death. Modern Mexicans still try to honor and comfort the dead by holding fiestas on All Soul's Day (November 2), popularly known in Mexico as the Day of the Dead.

Cultural views

Ancient cultures spent much time and effort on adequately preparing the dead for their journey to the afterlife, and they also had extremely precise views as to the appearance of this ultimate realm.

The Greek writer Plutarch recorded his understanding of what the next world would be like: "At first one wanders...through the dark...then come all the terrors before the final initiation: there is shuddering, a trembling, sweating,

---

Cinerary urn
This panel is part of an urn that held the ashes of an Etruscan couple cremated over 2,000 years ago. The panel shows the couple and attendants on their journey to the underworld.

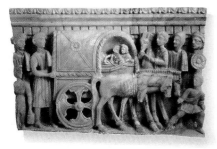

ASHES TO ASHES
Cremation was forbidden in Christian countries for centuries, but attitudes toward this practice began to change in the 19th century. Before modern systems of drainage were introduced, cemeteries represented a health hazard. In 1874 a group of doctors petitioned the Chamber of Deputies in Italy asking for the introduction of cremation. The Cremation Society of England was formed in the same year, but it was 1885 before the first publicly organized cremation took place. The Roman Catholic Church lifted its ban on the practice in 1964.

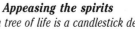
Appeasing the spirits
The Mexican tree of life is a candlestick decorated with birds, flowers, and angels, which is carried to cemeteries on the Day of the Dead.

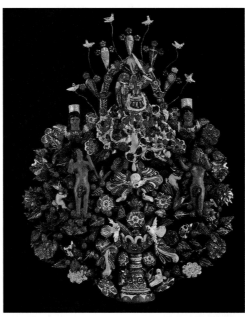

Marzipan skull
Colorfully decorated skulls made from marzipan are sold at fiestas on the Mexican Day of the Dead.

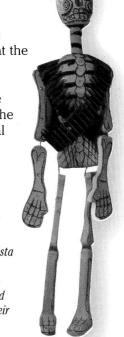

Honoring the dead
Papier maché skeletons and skulls are paraded in the streets during the annual fiesta for the Mexican Day of the Dead. Mexicans pray for the souls of departed friends and relations to help them in their transition to the next world.

amazement; then one is struck with a marvelous light, one is received into pure regions and meadows."

One early Christian description of the afterworld is found in the medieval saga *The Vision of Tundale*, written by an Irish monk who lived in Germany in the 12th

---

> # "Then one is struck with a marvelous light, one is received into pure regions and meadows."
> ### Plutarch

---

century. In a trance, the knight Tundale passed through a magic door into a lovely meadow crowded by sweet-smelling flowers. In the meadow stood the fountain of youth and a wall of silver. Beyond the wall Tundale saw souls in white robes giving thanks to God

Adorned at death
The Royal Cemetery of Ur consists of graves at the bottom of deep shafts. These were found to contain intact skeletons adorned with gold and semiprecious stones. Other exquisite objects, including golden cups, decorated vases, and ornate animal figures, such as the gold and lapis lazuli bull and goat seen here, were also buried within the stone chambers.

around a large tree full of blossoms, fruit, and birds. This was the tree of eternal life from the Garden of Eden.

Heavenly rewards

Many cultures came to believe that a suitable burial alone did not guarantee passage to a blissful afterlife. For a departed soul the greatest test was yet to come — their earthly lives had to undergo a godly assessment. The

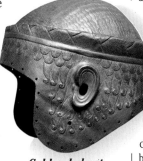

Golden helmet from Ur

verdict of this ultimate judgment resulted in an eternity of bliss or damnation. The Egyptian *Book of the Dead* introduced the idea that when people die, their treatment in an afterlife depends on their behavior on earth. According to the *Book of the Dead*, Egyptians of noble or

---

> # The possibility of a terrifying punishment in the afterlife is very real to many people.

---

royal birth, or people who had been especially brave or good during their lives, received their reward in the next world. This concept of judgment is now found in many religions.

Good and evil

The possibility of a terrifying punishment in the afterlife is very real to many people. The idea of hell originated in Persia (now Iran). Zoroaster, the ancient Persian religious leader who founded the Parsee religion in the sixth century B.C., viewed the world in terms of a constant struggle between the opposing forces of good and evil. Zoroaster's followers believe that the soul meditates on its life for three days

ROYAL CEMETERY

The Royal Cemetery of Ur was created by the great Sumerian civilization of Mesopotamia (3500-539 B.C.). The cemetery, which dates from about 2500 B.C., was discovered in the 1920's by British archeologist Sir Leonard Woolley.

Orderly departure

When the cemetery was opened up, archeologists discovered the remains of soldiers and women of the court. These attendants had been buried with their noble masters and mistresses in order to serve them in the afterlife. The fact that the attendants' bodies were found in orderly rows suggests that they went willingly to their deaths.

TAKING IT WITH YOU

The Chinese buried clothes, beds and bedding, money, and even live horses with a corpse for its use in the next world. As a result, burials were extremely expensive for the living, but even the poor did not want to risk angering a spirit of the dead by not carrying out these costly rituals.

Gradually, however, it became the custom to substitute paper effigies for the real items. This is still the practice in Hong Kong, where paper televisions, motorcars, and fake paper money are burned outside the homes of the dead.

Preparing paper effigies for a funeral in Hong Kong

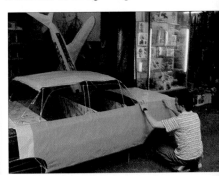

after death. The soul is then judged by the Wise Lord, Ahura Mazda, on the basis of all the good and evil thoughts, words, and deeds it has been responsible for in its life on earth. If good behavior has prevailed during an earthly life, a beautiful maiden leads the soul across a bridge to heaven. If evil deeds have dominated, an ugly old hag starts to take the soul across the bridge, but it falls off into hell. The soul's stay in either heaven or hell lasts until another day of resurrection when it is judged once again. Zoroaster's teachings influenced early Christian ideas about hell.

Route to rebirth
Buddhists and Hindus believe that the soul returns to earth in a series of lives. After death, souls go to the hall of the ruler of the dead where they are judged. Before rebirth in this world, most souls receive a temporary reward or punishment in heaven or hell, but some may stay in heaven or hell, never to return to earth. Hindus believe each human's essential self, or soul, can separate from the body. This self reincarnates in a series of bodies, human or animal, depending on behavior in a previous life. Early reference to this idea of souls moving between bodies, known as *samsara*, first appeared in Hindu literature in the 7th century B.C. According to Hindu belief the essential self suffers from the delusion that a life in an earthly body is desirable. Only through the knowledge gained during successive reincarnations can the notion of personal immortality be overcome. The self then merges into Brahman — the whole of the universe.

A similar concept appears in Buddhist thought. The Buddhist's ideal state of enlightenment is called *nirvana*. In the state of *nirvana*, all individual actions and personality are finally extinguished.

The Christian goal of meeting God in heaven does not require the loss of personal identity. Nor does Christianity accept the concept of reincarnation, regarding both heaven and hell as permanent realms.

A matter of fate
However, a belief in judgment is not universal. The citizens of ancient Mesopotamia believed that all people experienced exactly the same fate following death: To spend eternity in a dark, ghastly underworld where a person's rank or

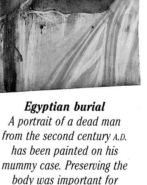

Egyptian burial
A portrait of a dead man from the second century A.D. has been painted on his mummy case. Preserving the body was important for survival in an afterlife.

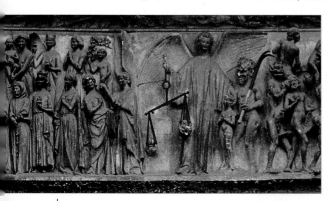

Scales of justice
This ancient Egyptian papyrus shows a dead person's heart being weighed against a feather. The figure adjusting the scale is Anubis, one of the gods of death.

DESTINIES IN BALANCE
From about 1600 B.C., Egyptians believed that the dead were judged in the Hall of Two Truths. The dead person's heart, which symbolized the conscience, was weighed against a feather that represented order and truth. If the heart weighed the same as the feather, the dead person lived happily in the afterlife. Those whose hearts proved too heavy fell victim to a monster that was part crocodile, part lion, and part hippopotamus. This creature was called the Eater of the Dead.

Christian judgment
A Christian version of the scales of judgment appears on this 13th-century stone relief from the cathedral in Bourges, France.

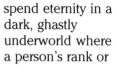

Wooden models
Ancient Egyptians believed there was work to be done in the afterlife. Wooden figures, like these models of bakers, brewers, and butchers were put in the tombs to do the labor. Magic spells inscribed on the figures brought them to life in the next world.

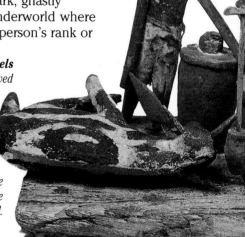

Root of power
People in some cultures believe that licorice, the sweet root of the blue-flowering pea, prolongs life and gives strength. The Egyptians, for example, believed the root would equip the newly dead with the power to ward off evil spirits. Small pieces of licorice root were found in Tutankhamun's tomb.

achievement did not count. In Polynesia, a person's good and evil deeds on earth make no difference to the ultimate fate of a soul after its death.

Ancestral power
For some cultures, such as the Aborigines of Australia and the Ashanti of West Africa, real knowledge and power can only be obtained in the spirit world and the respected dead are eventually worshiped as gods by the living. It is vital that the spirit of a dead person be happy with how it is being honored, otherwise it will seek revenge, so the living hold rituals to appease any vengeful dead. If kept content, the spirits could be very helpful. For example, Melanesians thought that their dead forebears appeared as birds to lead fishermen to abundant schools of fish.

Ideal location
Throughout our history the possibility that "something" leaves the body at death and continues to exist has been a constant preoccupation. Different cultures have developed detailed, and often opposing, views on the matter. The ideal way of preparing for the afterlife, the structure of heaven and hell, and the

possibility of a judgment have all been extensively discussed and chronicled over the ages. Some societies have even specified particular locations for their continued existence. In Greek mythology the heavenly Isles of the Blessed are to be found "somewhere in the west." The Hindu heaven is near a legendary Mount Meru at the center of the universe, which is thought to be located north of the Himalayas. Although there is no agreement about the whereabouts of the next life, the two most common beliefs include a happy afterlife situated in the sky and an unhappy afterlife under the earth.

> # The two most common beliefs include a happy afterlife in the sky and an unhappy afterlife under the earth.

To confirm the existence, structure, and location of the next world once and for all we would have to establish contact with the deceased themselves. Impossible as this task might seem, members of the spiritualist movement, formed in the 1850's, claim extensive and informative communication with the dead. The detailed and graphic descriptions of the afterlife that are supplied by spiritualist communicators contain some uncanny similarities with many ancient religious concepts.

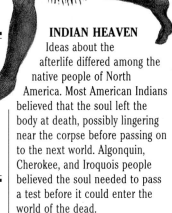

Algonquin medicine man

INDIAN HEAVEN
Ideas about the afterlife differed among the native people of North America. Most American Indians believed that the soul left the body at death, possibly lingering near the corpse before passing on to the next world. Algonquin, Cherokee, and Iroquois people believed the soul needed to pass a test before it could enter the world of the dead.

Sioux beliefs
The dead were feared by most American Indian groups, but not by the Sioux. Their funeral customs were devised to help the soul pass smoothly to the afterlife. Ideas about this next life were vague, but generally reflected what happened on earth. For example, a bountiful hunting ground after death was a common image for the native Americans of the prairies.

Several souls
The Inuit of northern Canada and Alaska believe that people have several souls, which are only temporarily associated with the body. The "free soul" lives on in another world after death and may return as a ghost. The "life soul" animates the body and dies with it.

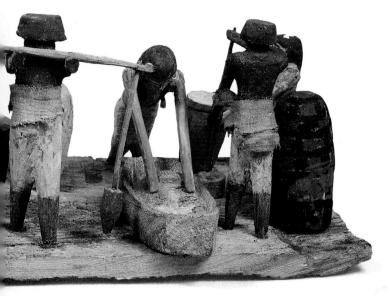

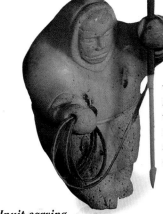

Inuit carving

THE SPIRITUALIST ADVENTURE

The world's ancient holy books contain many vivid descriptions of heaven and hell, but are they accurate predictions of what life after death is really like? Through spiritualist mediums, spirit communicators have provided startling images of the hereafter.

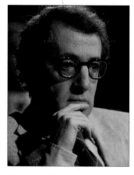

Woody Allen

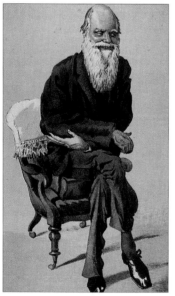

Charles Darwin

"O THIS IS DEATH!...I am at peace...I no longer need to strive and struggle, as I did in the earth life....As I look back over my earth life, I realize that so much was illusion."

"How does it feel to be 'dead?' One can't explain, because there's nothing in it. I simply feel free and light. My being seems to have expanded....After you die the soul suddenly seems to expand."

"As soon as I was able to bring myself to a conscious state of mind after my withdrawal from my worn-out body, I knew I was the same in essence."

These are just some of the many reports that mediums say they have received from people who have died and passed over to "the other side." Spirit communicators make contact with the living through psychics who claim to be in touch with a dimension beyond this life. Such receptive psychics, or mediums, often follow the ideas of spiritualism.

The astral view

Western spiritualism accepts several fundamental Christian principles: the Fatherhood of God, the Brotherhood of Man, the principle of personal responsibility (with reward or retribution in the life hereafter), the communion of spirits, the ministry of angels, continuous existence, and a path of endless progress leading toward the ultimate goal of universal salvation. The emphasis is on building good character and on love in its widest sense.

The spiritualist view is that within each individual's physical body resides an astral body that survives death. During life the astral body, a kind of ghostly double made of "subtle matter," coexists with the physical body. Spiritualists believe that during life, this astral body can separate from the

GRECO-ROMAN VIEW

The spiritualist view that some part of each individual survives death has its roots in ideas that are many centuries old. The ancient Greek poet Homer regarded death as destroying both the body and the conscious self. He considered that the only element to survive death was a phantom that went to an underground kingdom ruled by Pluto, the god of the dead, and his queen, Persephone. In this kingdom the dead moved as mere ghosts of themselves, away from laughter, love, and the joys of life.

The chosen ones

Homer's ideas represented the earliest view of the afterlife held by the Greeks. A belief developed from this that select people were allowed a blissful afterlife close to the gods. The notion of receiving rewards and punishments after a judgment became widespread.

The Greek philosopher Plato (427-347 B.C.) thought that possession of a soul is what distinguishes man from animals. An old man in Plato's *Republic*

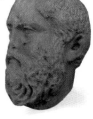

Plato

remarks that while death appears to be far away it is easy to laugh off tales of the underworld. As death becomes imminent, the old man wakes up in terror, fearing that tales of beatings by savage, fiery creatures in the afterlife may be true.

Roman underworld

The Roman poet Virgil (70-19 B.C.) described an underworld in his epic poem, the *Aeneid*. The poem's hero Aeneas goes into a cave and wanders in darkness until he finds the door to the land of the dead. There he encounters phantom monsters. He reaches a river where souls wait to be ferried across. On the other side a road divides, with a right path leading to paradise and a left path to a place where the wicked are horribly tortured.

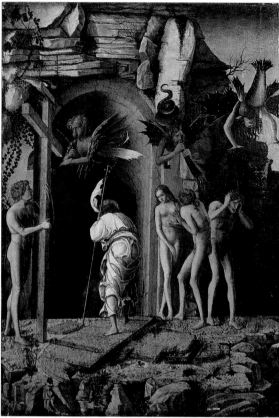

State of limbo
This painting by Giovanni Bellini (1429-1516) is entitled the "Descent into Limbo." Some Christian beliefs suggest that those who have not been baptized will spend eternity in limbo, which is neither heaven nor hell.

JUST REWARDS

Early Christians believed that after death every person received whatever treatment God judged appropriate. Those who didn't believe in Christ would suffer an eternity of hellish torture.

The "other place"

The Apocalypse of Peter, written in the second century, describes how Christ showed St. Peter paradise and then the "other place" where angels in dark robes tortured sinners. Adulterers were hung upside down over boiling muck while murderers were smothered by worms and other creeping creatures.

Heavenly route

Christian thought eventually evolved a clear-cut structure for the afterlife. Martyrs and good Christians would go directly to heaven while nonbelievers and the wicked went to hell. Those who were only slightly sinful went to an intermediate level called purgatory. Babies who had not been baptized went to limbo, a bland realm without the tortures of hell or the blessings of heaven. In the Christian ideal, there is no pain in heaven, no ugliness, and certainly no conflict.

physical body either consciously or unconsciously. People who have had near-death experiences often remember floating above their own bodies and watching the frantic attempts of medical staff to resuscitate them. These claims support the spiritualist concept of an astral body that can separate from the physical one, travel any distance and still be able to return.

Second sight

Although the astral body is considered by spiritualists to be invisible most of the time, there are several accounts of it being seen. In *The Techniques of Astral Projection,* author Robert Crookall recorded the case of Australian Lily Price. Ms. Price described the materialization of a young girl's astral body, "I saw a mist rise from the girl's head. The mist gradually took the shape of the child's bodily form." In 1980 *Theta* magazine published an

article by writer C. S Alvarado entitled "The Physical Detection of the Astral Body" which also described sightings of the astral body.

Spiritualists believe that the astral and physical bodies are linked by a silver cord that can stretch over any distance. Only at death does the cord break and the two bodies separate. This division was graphically described by Englishman Dr. R. B. Holt in the spiritualist journal *Light* in 1935. Dr. Holt was present at his aunt's deathbed, and

> ## "A silver-like substance...was streaming from the head of the physical body to the head of the spirit-double....At last the connecting strand snapped and the spirit-body was free."

as she died he said he saw, "A silver-like substance that was streaming from the head of the physical body to the head of the spirit-double. This cord seemed alive with vibrant energy....At last the connecting strand snapped and the spirit-body was free. The spirit-body, which had been supine before, now rose and stood vertically."

Another vivid account of the breaking of the cord that links the astral and the physical body appeared in a book entitled *Speaking Across the Borderline,* which was published in 1912. In the book Scotsman John Park verified many spiritualist teachings. What made the publication particularly interesting

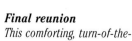

Final reunion
This comforting, turn-of-the-century image shows the dead meeting with lost friends and relatives.

was the fact that John Park had died several years before the book was written. During his life Park had been unconvinced by spiritualist ideas. However, following his death his wife, Fanny, reported receiving messages from him through the psychic powers of her aunt. Fanny felt that her husband's communications, which appeared in the form of automatic writing, were important enough to warrant publication. The resulting book contains Park's description of the gentle transition

> "Death does not take place until this cord has been severed. In most cases beloved arisen friends of the one who dies come about him to break this cord and bear him away."

from life to death: "Generally the spiritual counterpart floats horizontally above the dying form. It may remain for some time in this position, for it is attached to the body by a fine, filmy cord. Death does not take place until this cord has been severed. In most cases beloved arisen friends of the one who dies come about him at the last to break this cord and bear him away."

In his book *The Supreme Adventure*, Robert Crookall records numerous spirit messages, many of which suggest that even if a person has suffered greatly in the last moments of life, dying itself is

incredibly peaceful and free from pain. Death is a gradual withdrawal from the physical world, and is so natural that the transition to the spirit world can pass unnoticed. The astral self takes the form of an ideal version of the physical body that is as perfect as its owner can imagine it to be.

Shedding the physical body may be experienced as a momentary coma followed by a period of sleep, usually lasting a few days. Then comes the emergence into the next world. As one spirit communicator remarked: "Death really is just a sleep and an awakening."

New beginnings

In *The Supreme Adventure* Crookal cites messages purportedly from the dead that describe waking up with an expansion of consciousness. They speak of being greeted by friends and relations who have died previously: "When I woke completely I felt so refreshed...I knew I was not on earth, not only because of the long-lost people around me again, but because of the brilliancy of the atmosphere."

Mrs. Zoe Richmond, an author and a member of the Society for Psychical Research (SPR), believed that she had received a series of messages from her brother Joe, who had been killed during the First World War. SPR president Sir Oliver Lodge was particulary impressed by Joe's communications, writing that "There is a great deal of good matter in

HEAVEN ON EARTH
Swedish philosopher and religious writer Emanuel Swedenborg was born in Stockholm in 1688. He studied mathematics and science at the University of Uppsala and was by all accounts very down-to-earth as a young man. But in later life he reported experiencing some stunning glimpses of the afterlife.

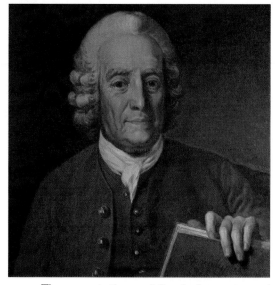

Emanuel Swedenborg

In 1743 Swedenborg started to have visions at night of angels and saints climbing what looked like heavenly staircases. He claimed that on the night of April 6, 1744, he had a face-to-face encounter with Christ.

Fate of the soul
Swedenborg believed that dying is simply a way in which the soul changes to another state.

According to Swedenborg, as a spirit arrives in the next world, it is received by angels. The spirit is then free to continue with a life very like the one it led previously while in the body.

Swedenborg died in London in 1772. After his death, various Swedenborgian religious societies were formed; these eventually merged to become the Church of the New Jerusalem.

Etruscan treasure
The Etruscans (800-200 B.C.) were the masters of central Italy before the ancient Roman Empire rose to power. Etruscans believed death led to a new existence in which people enjoyed the same pleasures as on earth. Much care was taken to build and decorate cemeteries. Possessions were buried with the dead for use in the afterlife.

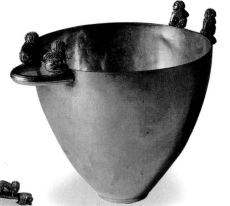

FREE SPIRITS

Before a traditional Hindu funeral ceremony, the corpse is washed, dressed, and decorated with jewels. The big toes and two thumbs are tied together to prevent any ghost of the dead person from returning to haunt the living. The corpse is then cremated. Hindus favor cremation as a method of disposing of the

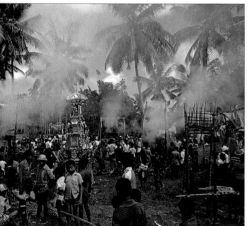

Hindu cremation grounds

dead because they believe the soul will linger near the physical body as long as it still exists. Burning the body allows the soul to take flight into the new body into which it is reincarnated.

Dangerous times

Despite these efforts, Hindus believe that some spirits and ghosts of the dead are still not at peace and keep trying to return to previous lives. The spirits are particularly dangerous at certain times of the year, such as late September or early October. Children are given special protection at this time so that they are not taken over by these spirits. Some Hindus put out daily offerings of food as appeasement.

them....So many people say that we get nothing of value, nothing about life on the other side...that really we ought to be able to show how false such statements are." According to Mrs. Richmond, Joe's messages described a new beginning: "After the sleep there is a difference....When the spirit comes out of that sleep he knows where he is and what he has become....The greater the difficulty of the spirit in adjusting himself to the new conditions, the longer and deeper the sleep period needed."

Familiar spirits

In other messages received by mediums the newly dead describe encounters with deceased loved ones as well as unfamiliar spirits who know all about them. One communication featured in Crookall's book described a meeting with one of these all-knowing spirits: "He regarded my whole life on earth — which hitherto I had thought of as being so important — as a mere preparation, a preliminary to the real work I have to do here. That has been one of the greatest surprises."

Communicators from the afterlife report through mediums that a human enters the next world with exactly the same character he or

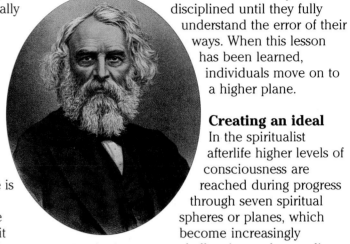

Poetic view
Poet Henry Wadsworth Longfellow (1807-82), who was also a professor at Harvard, summed up the spiritualist philosophy in "Resignation": "There is no death! What seems so is transition."

she had while living on earth. Those who have behaved badly are disciplined until they fully understand the error of their ways. When this lesson has been learned, individuals move on to a higher plane.

Creating an ideal

In the spiritualist afterlife higher levels of consciousness are reached during progress through seven spiritual spheres or planes, which become increasingly challenging and rewarding. The first plane is reported to be what you make of it, what you most desire. This is not "heaven," but "summerland." In this plane some souls seek to duplicate their home and possessions. One spirit may try to create an afterlife with the finest cigars and the best wines, while another may prefer to have a cup of coffee and comfortable rocking chair by an open fire. Two examples of individuals creating their own ideal in the afterlife can be found in messages reported by the English medium, Leslie Flint. The first of these communications was said to come from a coal miner who had been killed in a pit accident. He found himself on his back, lying in a meadow under bright sunshine. After a time he picked himself up and then walked across the field to an ideal cottage, which he knew to be his own. He was greeted by a dog, which he knew was his dog. He was feeling

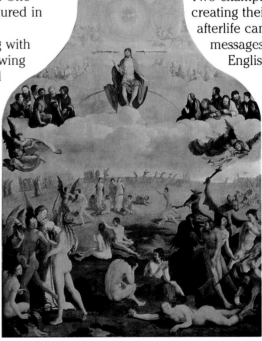

Help in the hereafter
"The Last Judgment" by Lucas van Leyden (c. 1494-1533). According to afterlife communicators, this final judgment is a highly enlightening experience which reveals all of the faults we have committed on earth.

completely content, he had everything he wanted. According to Flint the second message came from the great English stage actress Ellen Terry. She explained her increasing difficulty in maintaining contact with the earth-plane as she made progress through regions of indescribable beauty.

Spiritualists believe that in time souls learn that whatever they have created for themselves in the summerland is not spiritually rewarding, and that they are being too materialistic. The real purpose

> ## "My past deeds crowded before me. Oh, the anguish as deeds long-forgotten rose up.... nothing was forgotten."

of summerland is to help spirits realize that much of what they treasured during their lives is worthless.

For those who have led unsatisfactory lives and who have not considered the possibility of an afterlife, the realization of a continued existence can be far from pleasant. If there was no spiritual dimension to a person's life on earth, he or she may find him or herself lost in a kind of spiritual winterland, in a realm of gloom or fog, despondent and frustrated.

Acknowledging the afterlife
A selfish or a violent person may also end up in winterland, as his or her earthly behavior is a reflection of a poverty of the soul. But unbelieving or sinful spirits remain in winterland only as long as they refuse to acknowledge a higher part of themselves. Just as the concept of a summerland is not heaven, so a winterland is not hell. The belief is that both states are transcended when an individual matures spiritually. The lost soul is then rescued from winterland by helpful spirits. How long the process of self-discovery takes depends on how deeply the soul is tainted by its earthly desires and unworthy materialistic aims.

Judgment in the spiritualist afterlife is made not by God or some superior being. It is self-regulated, and based on a personal review of the earth life. Facing up to one's faults and errors results in a growing self-knowledge. Judging oneself is painful, but recognizing faults allows them to be transcended. In the afterlife the triviality of earthly priorities is seen with breathtaking clarity. In *The Supreme Adventure* spirits describe the painful experience of having their lives paraded before them:

"I was unconscious for a moment (when I shed my physical body), then my entire life unreeled itself."

"The first thing they find when they come here is the record of past life."

"I saw my life unfold before me in a procession of images."

"We are shown our mistakes and given a chance to alter and atone for all our wrongs."

"My past deeds crowded before me. Oh, the anguish as deeds that were long-forgotten rose up. Little or great, nothing was forgotten."

"I have been shown the effects of all my acts upon other people's minds. Their thoughts were shown to me. It was certainly the most humiliating and awful experience I have known."

Early spiritualist beliefs about the afterlife centered around the idea that life after death is experienced on a number of planes or spheres, formed in concentric circles, hundreds or thousands of miles above the earth. Today these planes are regarded as spiritual conditions with no particular geographic location. The planes are refined

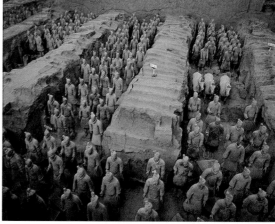

Terracotta army
Clay soldiers were buried to serve Chinese dead in the afterlife.

HAZARDOUS JOURNEYS
The Chinese believe that people have two souls, the hun soul, which is a spiritual and intellectual entity that passes on to heaven, and the more physical p'o soul, which follows the body into the grave or descends to a netherworld under the earth.

Chinese funeral rites aim to help the spirit of the hun soul join other hun souls in heaven, and to pacify the p'o to stop it from becoming a ghost. Traditionally, a valuable jewel was put in the mouth and buried with a Chinese corpse to honor the p'o soul to ensure that it felt well-treated by the living.

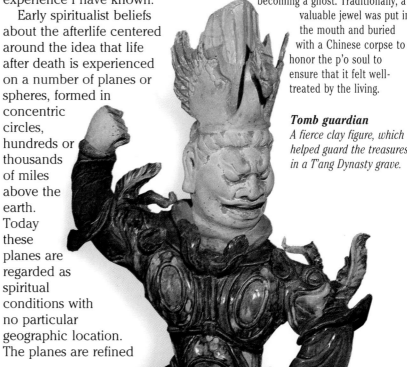

Tomb guardian
A fierce clay figure, which helped guard the treasures in a T'ang Dynasty grave.

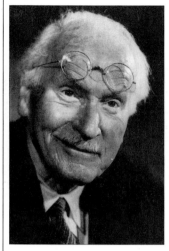

Carl Gustav Jung

COLLECTIVE UNCONSCIOUS
Swiss pychologist Carl Gustav Jung (1875-1961) introduced the idea of the collective unconscious. This is very like the pooled memory suggested by English physiologist Dr. Rupert Sheldrake. Jung felt that, at a conscious level, our individual minds are separated, but that our unconscious minds are merged, and linked to those who have lived before. This concept supports the theory that a collective memory for humankind may exist, which could make the experience of our ancestors available to us all.

states through which the spirit progresses on its long, searching journey to enlightenment.

Some psychics have suggested the possibility of a "second death," which allows the spirit to shed all that remains from the earthly world and puts it beyond earthly contact. It is only after this second death that someone can experience "second heaven" and

---

Individual spirits lose their limitations and evolve into a state of complete fusion beyond our earthly imagination.

---

progress further in the spiritual realm. When a spirit is ready, further expansion of consciousness in a "third heaven" is possible. And so the soul develops.

Moving on to the more spiritual levels beyond second and third death is possible only when a soul is able to appreciate a higher plane. There may be an ultimate sphere where individual spirits lose their limitations and evolve into a state of complete fusion beyond our earthly imagination. Spiritualists hold the view that spirits come together in the ascending spheres to form group souls. With advanced

spiritual development, these groups become permanent, each spirit making a unique contribution to a larger entity.

Belief in reincarnation has been a part of many religions and cultures, and spiritualism is no exception. Spiritualists suggest that as souls transcend the various spiritual planes of the afterlife, they come to realize that they have been reincarnated many times previously. In the afterlife past lives are seen as part of a pattern that has a purpose, and previous earth lives are seen as only a fragment of a much larger whole. Events in the latest earth life may well be the consequence of actions in previous lives. Wiser beings advise the soul on how to improve so that the next life on earth will be more informed and more spiritual. For spiritualists death offers the prospect of ever-expanding consciousness and the chance of new beginnings for us all.

Freedom from sin
Many strange rituals have been devised to help souls in the afterlife. Until the mid-1800's, it was common in Britain to hire an old man as a Sin Eater. He would take upon himself all the sins of the dead in exchange for sixpence, beer, and a loaf of bread that had been left next to the corpse. Traditionally, in Brittany, France, a pitcher of milk was placed near a dead body to "whitewash" it of sins before judgment day. The teachings of spiritualism suggest that fears for the soul are unnecessary, as the afterlife provides a learning experience without lasting punishment.

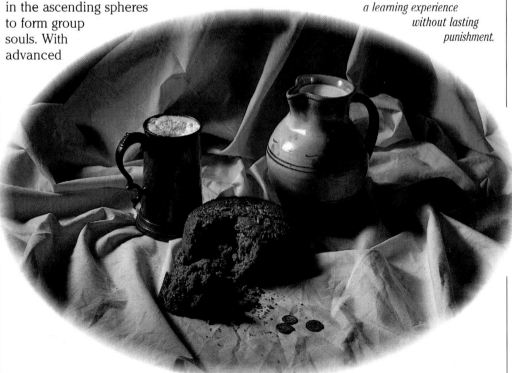

POOLED RESOURCES

Are messages from the dead the only way we can benefit from our ancestors' experience? Dr. Rupert Sheldrake, an English physiologist, thinks our predecessors share their collective wisdom in another, less personal way.

*I*N 1981 DR. RUPERT SHELDRAKE published a book called *A New Science of Life* which questioned many of the basic principles of Western science and caused an uproar in scientific circles. *Nature* magazine said that the book was "The best candidate for burning there has been for many years," while *World Medicine* magazine stated that "Wild as they seem, Sheldrake's ideas are difficult to refute." Sheldrake even appeared before the U.S. Congress to discuss his controversial theories.

Rupert Sheldrake studied natural sciences at Clare College, Cambridge, England, and philosophy and the history of science at Harvard. Between 1967 and 1973 he was director of studies in biochemistry and cell biology at Clare College. It came as a shock to Sheldrake's fellow academics when he suggested that they should put aside their conventional ideas about how the world works, and dismiss the scientific convention that the form and behavior of all things are governed by mere molecules.

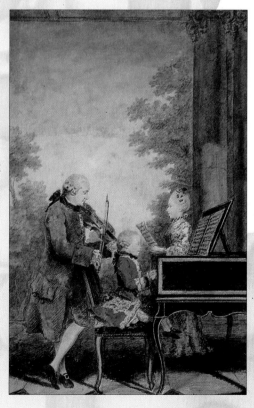

Dr. Rupert Sheldrake

The mystery of heredity

Even the most traditional biologists accept that there is a mysterious factor involved in heredity. It is a scientific fact that every cell in the body contains DNA, deoxyribonucleic acid, which is the basic carrier of genetic information. But within any one body, all cells have the same DNA structure and yet these cells develop into quite different limbs and organs. Science has yet to establish what determines this varied development. Dr. Sheldrake suggests that development is governed by "morphogenetic fields," which he describes as being a "new type of physical field which plays a role in the

Mystery of life
In 1953, at Cambridge University, James Watson and Francis Crick uncovered the structure of DNA and thereby made one of the great discoveries of modern science. The existence of DNA had been recognized since the mid-1800's, but no one realized that it carried the message of heredity. DNA is contained in long thread-like chromosomes wrapped around each other in a spiral, known as the double helix. Although much is now known about DNA, it is still not understood why cells develop differently when they all contain the same DNA.

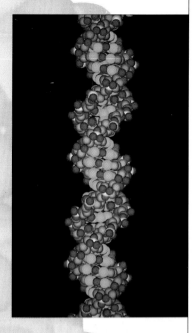

development of form." According to Dr. Sheldrake, it is these morphogenetic fields that help to mold the construction of cells and tissues.

Dr. Sheldrake believes that similar beings are linked across time and space by morphogenetic fields, and that these fields allow creatures to learn from previous members of the same species even when there has been no physical contact between them. Dr. Sheldrake says that when any animal learns a new form of behavior it will influence the subsequent learning of all animals of the same kind. We may be learning from those who have lived before us without realizing that we are doing so, and therefore it should become easier for people to learn new skills, simply because more and more people have acquired these skills in the past.

Although Sheldrake's work has been refuted by much of the conventional scientific world, it has certainly made a great impact. *Brain/Mind Bulletin* expressed the view that his concept was "as far reaching as Darwin's theory of evolution."

Child prodigy
Mozart was a child prodigy who began composing at the age of four. According to Dr. Sheldrake, such talent may have been gathered from other musicians.

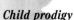

Visions of Heaven and Hell

Inspired by religious belief or personal insight, artists over the ages have fascinated us with haunting visions of both the terrors of damnation and the splendors of redemption.

THE IDEA OF A LAST JUDGMENT is found in many cultures. Those who have led decent lives receive rewards in the afterlife; those who have been evil are punished. Artists from different cultures and periods have attempted to describe the afterlife, often in remarkably similar terms.

One common vision shows heaven as a park or garden. The word *paradise* itself comes from the ancient name for the enclosed parks constructed for Persian kings. There is also a similarity between contemporary descriptions of the next world supplied by those who have "died" and then been resuscitated (a near-death experience), and centuries-old artistic interpretations of both heaven and hell.

The Dutch artist Hieronymus Bosch (1450-1516) has produced some of the most imaginative and detailed scenes of what might happen after we die.

Torment of the damned

For Bosch, damnation was mainly a physical agony. He depicted the torments explicitly. Naked bodies of the damned are shown mutilated, tortured, and gnawed at by serpents. Bosch also introduced strange animal-human combinations. In his paintings the orderly laws of nature have been replaced by chaos, in which the grotesque and the unnatural rule.

In Bosch's work some specific sins are readily identifiable. Bosch considered gambling, with its greed for monetary gain, among the worst types of ungodly behavior. In the bottom left corner of the "hell" panel of "The Garden of Earthly Delights," gamblers are shown with their hands cut off as a warning to the living. Although many artists have attempted to depict the perfection of heaven, it is often the harrowing images of hell that make the most powerful and lasting impressions on the viewer.

Belphegor — a biblical demon of evil

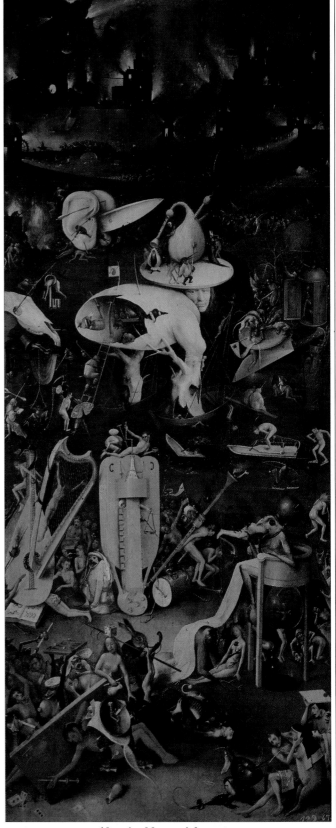

Abominable punishments
The "hell" panel of Hieronymus Bosch's "The Garden of Earthly Delights" is filled with repulsive images. One figure is helplessly ensnared in the strings of a giant harp. A huge pair of ears moves like a tank, attacking its victims with a great knife.

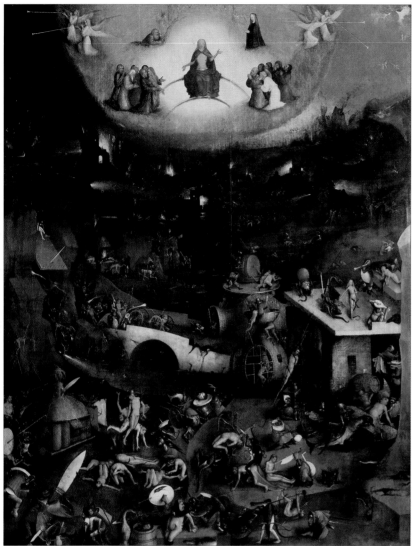

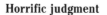

Horrific judgment

In this, the central panel of "The Last Judgment" by Bosch, a man is shown being roasted slowly on a spit, basted by a small ugly beast with a bloated belly. A female demon has sliced her victim like ham and is frying him to accompany the eggs shown at her feet. Other punishments are equally bizarre. A glutton is forced to drink from a barrel held by two devils, and the unpleasant contents are supplied by a figure squatting in the window above.

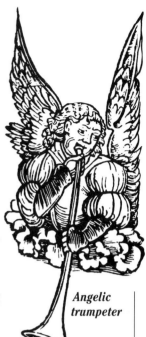

Angelic trumpeter

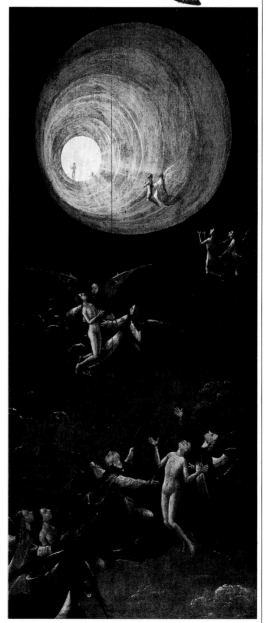

Demonic works

This demon was visualized by the German artist Hans Holbein the Younger (1497-1593).

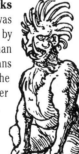

Hellish descent

Many artistic interpretations of hell show demonic creatures torturing the wicked, as they are in this gruesome painting by Dieric Bouts (1410-75).

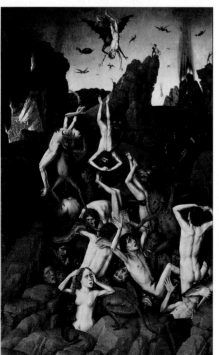

Heavenly ascent

"The Ascent into the Empyrean" by Hieronymus Bosch shows souls being taken up to heaven by angels. A very similar tunnel leading to a bright light has often been described in modern accounts of near-death experiences.

Buddhist heaven

Just as traditional Christian belief has divided heaven and hell into rings or layers, Eastern religions have a compartmentalized view of the afterworld. Some Buddhists believe there are eight major hells and no fewer than 128 lesser hells.

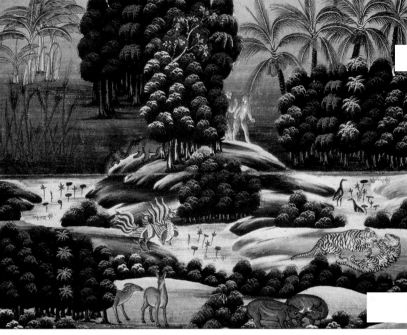

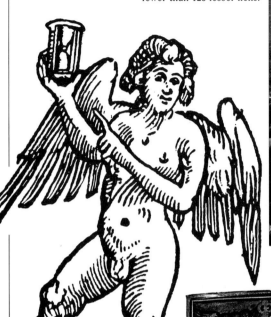

A winged angel of death with skull and hourglass

Consumed by fire

In this 14th-century French manuscript the entrance to hell is shown as two huge mouths. Christian art often shows the dead entering hell through the mouth of some animal or monster. This concept stems from an ancient fear of being devoured, a fate which was thought to deny a person any chance of happiness in the afterlife.

A devil drags a victim toward the fires of hell

Tortured flesh

This vision of hell by Italian artist Luca Signorelli (*c.* 1450-1523) was painted in the early 1500's. As in many other images, hell is filled with souls locked together in conflict. Heaven, on the other hand, is usually depicted as a serene, spacious domain.

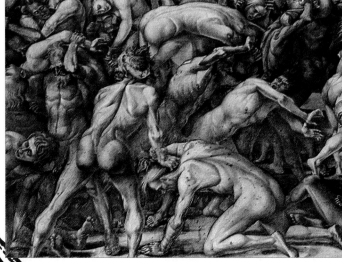

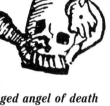

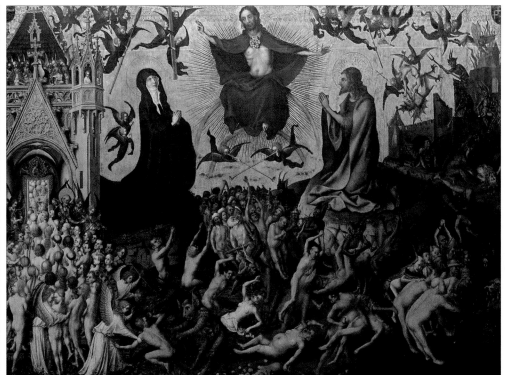

Divine justice
This early Renaissance interpretation of "The Last Judgment" was painted *c.* 1445 by German artist Stefan Lochner (1400-1451). Winged angels take fortunate souls to heaven, while the less fortunate are attacked by demons of unspeakable ugliness. The Last Judgment was a popular theme in medieval and early Renaissance art. The Christian church teaches believers how to behave if they wish to be blessed and avoid a sentence of eternal damnation.

Angelic pose
This 17th-century sculpture by Gian Lorenzo Bernini (1598-1680) shows the marvelous grace and beauty associated with heavenly angels.

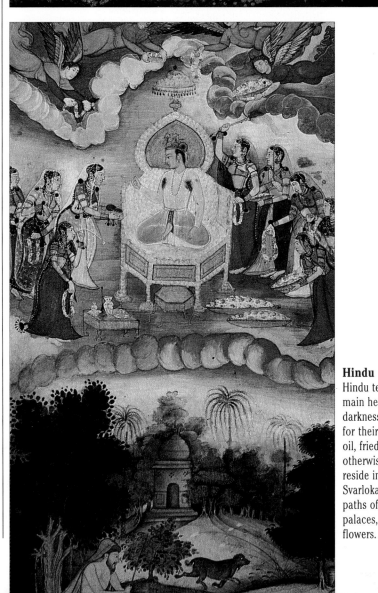

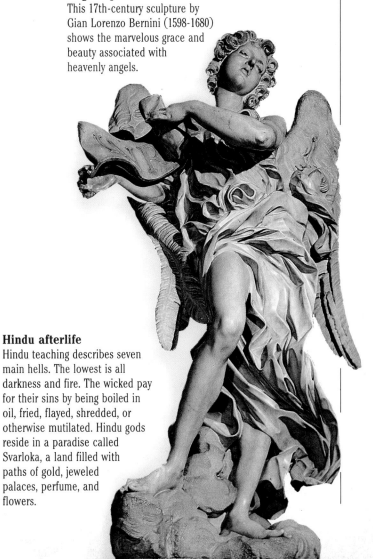

Hindu afterlife
Hindu teaching describes seven main hells. The lowest is all darkness and fire. The wicked pay for their sins by being boiled in oil, fried, flayed, shredded, or otherwise mutilated. Hindu gods reside in a paradise called Svarloka, a land filled with paths of gold, jeweled palaces, perfume, and flowers.

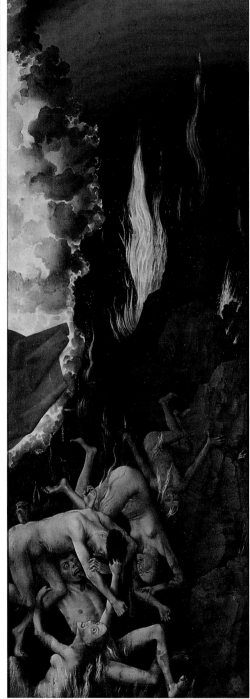

Lucifer devouring Judas

Modern comparisons

William Blake (1757-1827) was
an English poet and painter,
and also something of a
visionary. Many of his paintings
depict scenes of an afterlife,
supposedly revealed to him by
spirits. Some of the scenes are
very like modern descriptions of near-death experiences. The watercolor
"Jacob's Dream" portrays angels on a staircase moving heavenward.
The angels seem to be leading spirits toward a glowing light.

Burning desires

Rogier van der Weyden (1399-1464) showed the
wicked burning in the eternal fires of hell in one
panel of his painting "The Last Judgment." Fire is
prominent in many visions of the underworld.

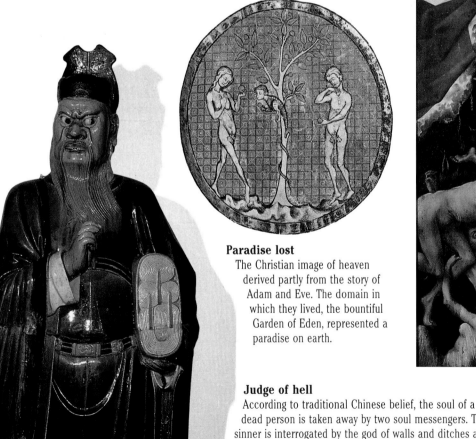

Paradise lost

The Christian image of heaven
derived partly from the story of
Adam and Eve. The domain in
which they lived, the bountiful
Garden of Eden, represented a
paradise on earth.

Judge of hell

According to traditional Chinese belief, the soul of a
dead person is taken away by two soul messengers. The
sinner is interrogated by the god of walls and ditches and
then by a series of judges. Each judge delivers a
punishment before passing the sinner on to the next judge.
The final judge of hell sends the sinner back to earth in a
form appropriate to his or her past crimes.

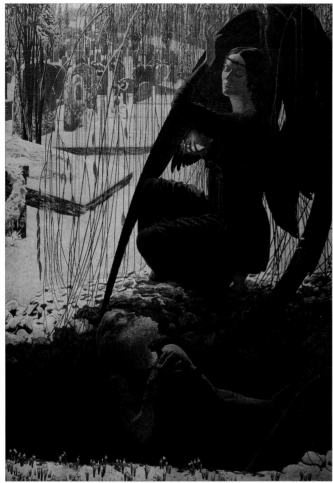

Deathly messenger
The Belgian painter Carlos Schwabe (1866-1926) portrayed "Death and the Gravedigger." Traditional Jewish belief holds that an angel of death arrives for each person when his or her time on earth ends.

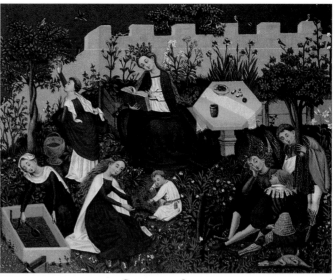

Serene garden
Many cultures visualize heaven as a garden, as in this 15th-century painting. The garden represents peace, beauty, and tranquility — an ideal far removed from the pressures of life on earth and the ghastly and unending tortures of hell.

Deadly sins
For Christians the consequence of committing any of the seven deadly sins is severe punishment. Pride, covetousness, lust, anger, gluttony, envy, and sloth can all result in final damnation. In this 15th-century French engraving the lustful are left to simmer painfully.

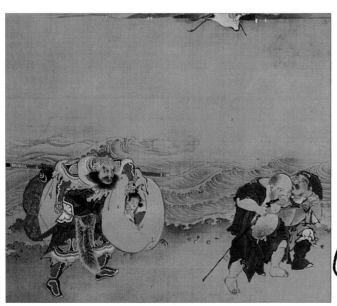

Warrior heaven
Shinto, the national religion of Japan until after the Second World War, promised a paradise such as this to those who were brave in battle and loyal to the emperor.

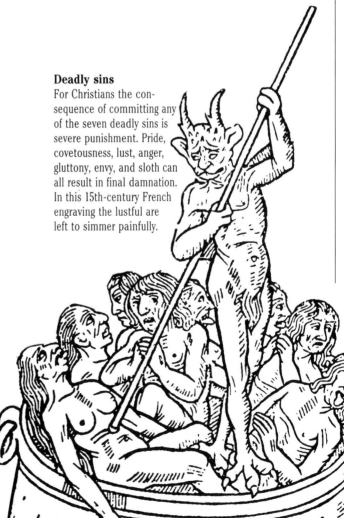

SURVIVAL PACTS

Agreeing, while still alive, on some signal, message, or clue that can be delivered after death is one way to test whether there is an afterlife. Such pacts are now being recorded in an effort to solve this enduring mystery.

IN 1882, DURING A DISCUSSION about spiritualism, two friends, Count Charles Galatéri and Lieutenant M. Virgini, made a pact that whoever died first would try to alert the other by tickling his feet. On the evening of Sunday, August 5, 1888, six years after the two men had made their agreement, Galatéri was lying in bed when his wife complained that her feet were being tickled. The couple could find nothing to explain the sensation, but the countess then exclaimed, "Look! Look at the foot of the bed....There's a tall young man, with a colonial helmet on his head. He's looking at you, and laughing! Oh, poor man! What a terrible wound he has in his chest! And his knee is broken! He's waving to you with a satisfied air. He's disappearing."

Decisive tests

The next day the countess told her friends about the experience and nine days later on Tuesday, August 14, Virgini's death in action in Abyssinia was reported in the press. He had been shot in the knee and then killed by a bullet in the chest. It was at about the time of his death that Virgini appeared to the Countess Galatéri and tickled her feet.

The above story, reported in an Italian journal of psychical research published in 1905, is just one of many examples of survival pacts. Friends agree that the first to die will try to contact the other after death in order to prove that existence continues. Some contacts from the dead have been reported, but there is still very little evidence to support the claims.

In 1903, F. W. H. Myers, one of the founders of the Society for Psychical Research (SPR), wrote in his book entitled *Human Personality and its Survival of Bodily Death:* "I think it very desirable that as many people as possible should provide a decisive test of their identity in case they should find themselves able to communicate through any sensitive after their bodily death." Before his death, Myers left a written message in a sealed envelope, with a view to communicating its secret contents after his death. The drawback of such a test was that only one trial could be made. Once the envelope had been opened, its contents would no longer be unknown.

A more impressive result of a survival-pact experiment was described to Richard Hodgson, SPR

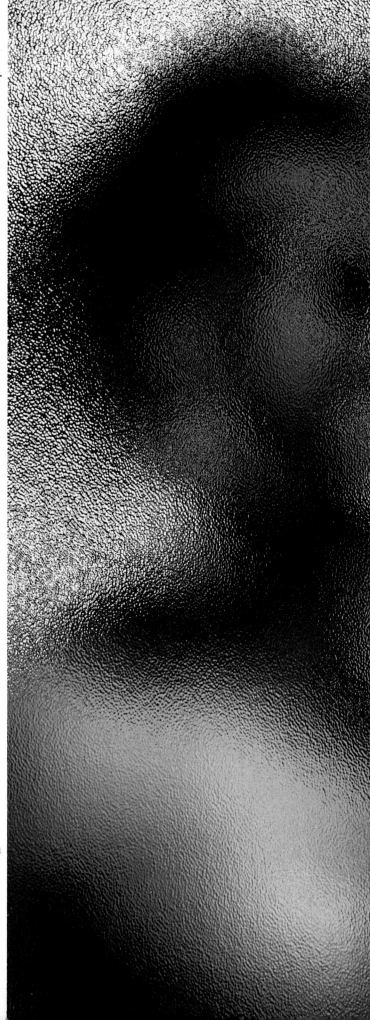

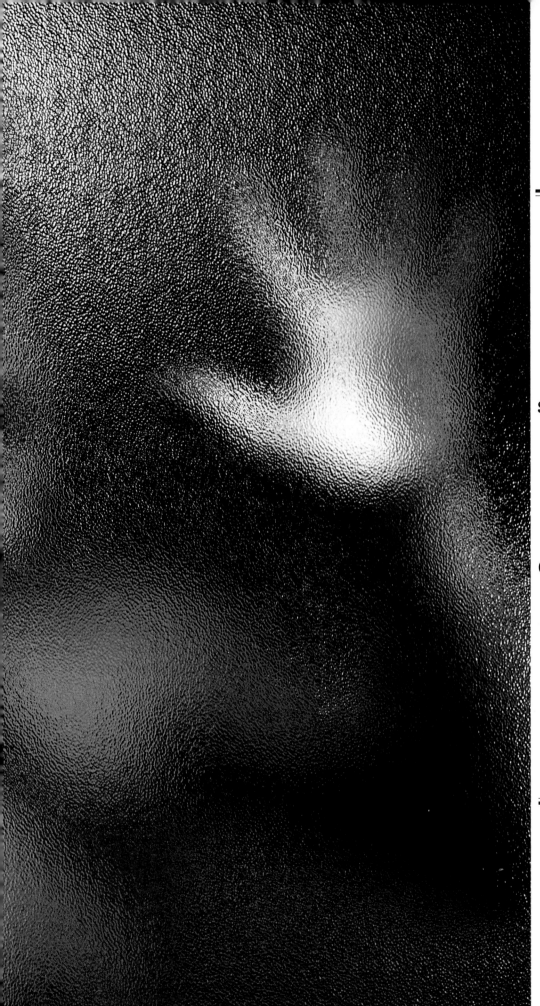

"The nearest simile I can find to express the difficulties of sending a message is that I appear to be standing behind a sheet of frosted glass — which blurs sight and deadens sounds — dictating feebly to a reluctant and somewhat obtuse secretary."

F. W. H. Myers speaking through the automatic writing of a medium in 1906, five years after his death, as reported in *Proceedings,* Society for Psychical Research, Vol. XXI

RAPPING MESSAGES

The dead seem to honor their survival pacts by various means. One technique has been called table-rapping. This was very popular in the mid-1800's in Britain, North America, France, Germany, Turkey, and China. The technique involves participants sitting around a table, their fingertips resting lightly on the surface and touching those of their neighbors on either side.

Lengthy messages

Questions are asked of the spirit world and the table responds by rapping one or more legs on the floor. One rap is usually considered to mean "yes," two raps means "uncertain," and three raps from the table leg means "no." The table may spell out words by using a different number of raps for each letter of the alphabet. One tap would be *A*, two taps for *B*, and so on to the letter *Z*. In this way, a message from the afterlife may be communicated. Spelling out long messages may sound tedious today, but groups found this to be exciting entertainment before the advent of cinema, radio, and television.

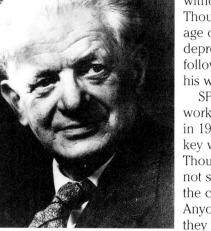

Legs tapping

This illustration shows unexpected events at a fashionable London séance of the 1870's.

American representative, by a Mrs. Finney of Rockland, Massachusetts, in 1891. As Mrs. Finney explained, her cousin Benja marked one half of a small brick with ink and gave his sister the other half. Benja hid his part of the brick and promised to reveal its whereabouts if he died first.

After Benja's death in 1866, a message did come to the family during a table-rapping session. Each set of raps corresponded to a letter of the alphabet. The message, slowly spelled out in this way, said: "You will find that piece of brick in the cabinet under the tomahawk. Benja." The brick was found concealed in a cabinet that had not been opened since Benja's death. Benja also sent another message that corresponded exactly with one he had left in a sealed envelope: "Julia — do right and be happy — Benja."

Dr. Robert Thouless, a SPR member, devised another type of test in 1948. The test consisted of two coded sequences: INXPH CJKGM JIRPR FBCVY WYWES NOECN SCVHE CYRJQ TEBJM TGXAT TWPNH CNYBC FNXPF LFXRV QWQL and BTYRR OOFLH KCDXK FWPCZ KTADR GFHKA HTYXO ALZUP PYPVF AYMMF SDLR UVUB. After his death Dr. Thouless intended to communicate the keys to decipher the sequences. The only clues were that the key to the first is a continuous passage of poetry or prose, while the key to the second sequence consisted of just two words. Thouless challenged mediums to read

Distinguished researcher

Dr. Robert Thouless was a distinguished psychologist and parapsychologist. He was a Reader Emeritus at Cambridge University, England, and published a number of books and articles. Besides being past president of the Society for Psychical Research, Thouless was associated with the Parapsychology Laboratory at Duke University and its successor, the Foundation for Research on the Nature of Man.

the keys from his mind while he was still alive. He argued that if this could not be done while he was alive, but *could* be done after his death, this would prove the definite existence of an afterlife. In 1948 and 1949 the SPR enlisted mediums to read the key words from Thouless's mind, without success. Thouless died at the age of 90 in 1984, in a depressed state of mind following the death of his wife.

SPR members worked with mediums in 1985 to retrieve the key words from Thouless. The test did not succeed. However, the case is still open. Anyone who thinks they may have received the clue that will unlock either of Dr. Thouless's messages should contact the Society for Psychical Research at 49 Marloes Road, London W8 6LA, England.

Prof. Ian Stevenson of the University of Virginia has also devised a test, using a combination lock. The purchaser of a combination lock sets it to numbers that he or she keeps secret. A word clue to the numbers, such as a rhyme, is decided. After the person's death, mediums attempt to read the clue to the numbers. The odds against this clue being found by chance are 1 in 125,000.

Communication — or coincidence?

In 1963 a Survival Joint Research Committee used a number of combination locks to set up an experiment to promote cooperation between psychical researchers and spiritualists. However, by the 1990's no locks left by deceased members of the committee had been opened. If spiritualists are correct, the deceased are frantically trying to honor their pacts — but few of us have the psychic ability to hear them.

CONCLUSIVE COMMUNICATIONS

"The departed spirit should be trying to communicate something which could not be known to mediums by any psi process, and it should be something seen as right when it comes however many false attempts have been made."
Dr. Robert Thouless

AN INTRIGUING EXERCISE is to devise a test for the reality of life after death. Could you and your friends invent a test now that would confirm an afterlife if one exists? Such pacts as have been made to date have met with little or no success. But organizations have now been set up worldwide to advise and assist those who hope to provide conclusive proof of the existence of an afterlife.

Afterlife experiences

There is growing support for the view that death is not the end of conscious existence. For example, in 1990 The International Association for Near-Death Experiences published a survey of 300 NDE subjects. Many of these people had been pronounced clinically dead and then "came back" to life. Half of the subjects surveyed said that their experiences had convinced them that there is an afterlife. The idea of survival pacts is to provide some kind of concrete proof for a life after death, if it does in fact exist.

Here are a few suggestions for your own survival pact:

◆ Padlock
Devise a clue that could be sent from the afterlife to open a padlock.

◆ Sealed envelope
Leave a message in a sealed envelope, and pass on its contents psychically if there is a next world.

◆ Code
Create a code that can only be solved by clues communicated after death.

Recording the pact

An important part of any pact you make is to record the details, and any results, with an outside source. Researchers hope that, in time, enough material will be collected to establish if there is a life after death. An organization involved in this study is the Survival Research Foundation, P.O. Box 8565, Pembroke Pines, Florida 33024. The SRF organizes cipher, lock, and other tests, and records individual pacts.

INXPH CJKGM JIRPR
FBCVY WYWES NOECN SCVHE
CYRJQ TEBJM TQXAT TWPNH
CNYBC FNXPF LFXRV QWQL

FAMOUS LAST WORDS

People about to die may utter significant last words before learning the ultimate secret puzzling humankind. Is death the end or merely the beginning of a new existence? Here is a selection of some last, dying words. Do they offer any vital clues for the living?

◆ *"In my end is my beginning."*
*Mary, Queen of Scots,
executed 1587.*

*H*UMANKIND FACES DEATH in many moods. Some people believe it represents the absolute end of existence – while others feel it is the start of a new adventure either in heaven or hell, or in another reincarnation on earth. Whether the dying are fearful or relieved, reluctant or resigned, their final words have a certain poignancy for those who have yet to discover the greatest mystery of the unknown.

◆ **"Why fear death? It is the most beautiful adventure in life."**
Charles Frohman, drowned when the S.S. Lusitania *was torpedoed in 1915.*

◆ **"How grand is the sunlight."**
Friedrich Humbolt, German traveler and scientist, died 1859.

◆ **"I see the black light!"**
Victor Hugo, French poet, died 1885.

Victor Hugo

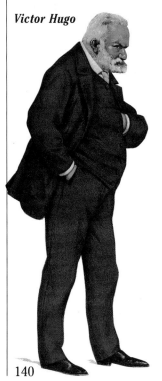

◆ **"What does it matter? They may kill the body, but they cannot kill the soul."**
Huldrych Zwingli, Swiss reformer, killed 1531.

◆ **"I have had a beautiful vision, a beautiful vision."**
Theodore Thomas, orchestra conductor, died 1905.

◆ **"If I had the strength to hold a pen, I would write how easy and pleasant it is to die."**
William Hunter, professor of anatomy, died 1783.

◆ **"I shall look forward to a pleasant time."**
John Hancock, signatory of the Declaration of Independence, died 1793.

John Hancock

"It is very beautiful over there."
Thomas Alva Edison, inventor, died 1931.

"This is not the end of me."
Sir Henry Campbell-Bannerman, British prime minister, died 1908.

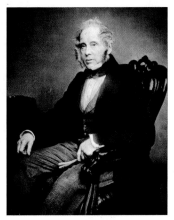

Lord Palmerston

"Die, my dear doctor? That's the last thing I shall do!"
Lord Palmerston, British prime minister, died 1865.

"Six feet of earth for my body and the infinite heavens for my soul is what I shall soon have."
Anne du Bourg, French martyr, executed 1559.

"Oh, I hear such beautiful voices."
Mary-Anne Schimmelpenninck, author of children's books, died 1856.

"Oh Mother, how beautiful it is."
Cholly Knickerbocker, New York gossip columnist, died 1942.

"There is another and a better world."
John Palmer, British actor, died on stage in 1798 after saying these words.

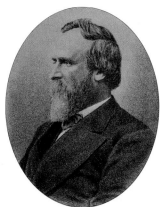

Rutherford B. Hayes

"I know that I'm going where Lucy is."
Rutherford B. Hayes, American president, died 1893, welcoming the chance to see his wife, Lucy, again.

AFTERLIFE REPORTING

Perhaps the words of the dying give us a brief insight into the next world. However, in some cases, like that of the famous British adventurer Lawrence of Arabia, the deceased may be able to provide a more detailed description.

THOMAS EDWARD LAWRENCE (1888-1935), British archeologist and soldier, was called Lawrence of Arabia following his dramatic adventures in the desert during the First World War.

Jane Sherwood, a British medium, claims that Lawrence communicated his after-death experiences through her. Sherwood had found herself questioning the purpose of life and the possibility of life after death, following the death of her husband, Andrew, during the Second World War. She began to read spiritualist literature, attend séances, and consult with mediums. Finally, she started to receive communications, in the form of automatic writing, which she believed to be from the spirit world. The story of her acceptance of spiritualism was told in her first book, *The Psychic Bridge.* Subsequent titles, *The Country Beyond* and *Fourfold Vision*, contained the scripts of her various automatic communications.

In 1964 Sherwood published a book called *Post-Mortem Journal*, which chronicled the communications she claimed to have received from T. E. Lawrence. In the book Lawrence is said to describe how, soon after death, everything was reduced to a monochrome. There was no sound, no movement, no light, and no joy. He felt at first that it might have been better if his life had indeed ended at death.

He did not know how long this "weary experience" lasted. He was then taken by a new friend through an ever-brightening

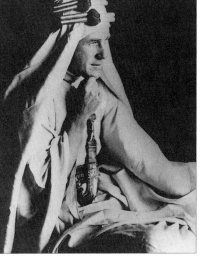

Arab costume
T. E. Lawrence was a British adventurer who felt a particular affinity with Arab culture.

landscape. The friend explained that Lawrence's senses had to be given time to adjust to the new world, and that the new world would hold only what Lawrence was capable of seeing in it.

Lawrence began to miss the weight of his earth body, and he found himself moved by powerful pangs of emotion that were almost impossible to control. These emotions were not the inward things they were on earth. He likened the strength of his emotions to driving a fast, powerful car when someone has been used to a slow vehicle. He disliked the insecurity, but felt exhilarated.

According to Jane Sherwood, Lawrence said that in paradise there are noble buildings, as well as stretches of lovely countryside with parks and mansions, "wild regions of mountain and moor and rivers and seas of incomparable beauty." There is no need to produce and consume food, and there are no extremes of temperature. "When people first arrive here the ease with which any desired goods can be obtained sometimes goes to their head. They clutch and hoard as they would have done on earth; but this is usually a temporary phase."

Ageless existence
One intriguing aspect of the afterlife reported by Sherwood is the way people whose earth lives were separated by centuries are able to coexist. Lawrence pointed out that he was associating with his grandfather, great-grandfather, and others going back for generations — yet they were all roughly the same age in the next life, "One gets a mixture of the manners and customs of many ages and historical eras."

According to Jane Sherwood's book, there is a chance for progress in the afterlife, people move to a higher plane as their spiritual development justifies it.

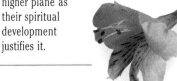

INDEX

Page numbers in **bold** type refer to illustrations and captions.

A

Aborigines, 42, 121
Adam and Eve, **134**
Aeneid (Virgil), 123
Aetherius Society, 88
Africa, 106, 115, 121
Akashic Records, 54
Alaska, 61, 121
Albigensians, 46, **46**
Algonquin, 121, **121**
Allen, Woody, 122, **122**
Alvarado, C. S., 124
Andrew Bobola, St., 99, 100
Angels, 65, **131, 132, 133**
Angkor Thom, temple carvings, 42
Annaya, Lebanon, 101
Anti-vampire devices, 113-114, **113, 114**
Apocalypse of Peter, The, 124
Apparitions, **75, 88,** 90, 91-92, **92,** 93, 94, **94,** 95, **95**
   crises, 96-97
Arnaud, F. L., 68
Ars, France, **101**
Art, psychic, 76, 82, 84, **85**
"Ascent into the Empyrean, The" (H. Bosch), **131**
Astral travel, 34, **34,** 38, **38-39,** 86
Astrology, **60, 61,** 70-71, **70-71**
Atlantis, 55, **70-71,** 71
Augustine, St., 45, 46
Awakenings (Dr. O. Sacks), 111

B

Ba, Bird of Death, **39**
Bacon, Francis, **71,** 122
Balfour, Arthur James, **81**
Balfour, Gerald W., **80,** 81
Bali, Indonesia, 46, 65, **65**
Bangs, Lizzie & May, 76, **76**
Bannerjee, Hemendra, 48, 59
Bara, Theda, **112**
Baron Samedi, 115
Barrett, Sir William, 76, 91
Bastos, Judge Orimar de, 83
Bathory, Countess E., 114, **114**
Bat, vampire, **114**
Bayless, Raymond, **82,** 83
Belasco, David, 96-97
Belief in a Life After Death, The (C. J. Ducasse), 77
Bellini, Giovanni, **124**
Belphegor, demon of evil, **130**
Berlin, 101, **111**
Bernini, Gian Lorenzo, **133**
Bernstein, Dr. Morey, 50, 53, 54
Berruguete, Pedro, **46**
Bey, Rahman, **106**
Beyond Biofeedback (E. & A. Green), 109
Biegas, Boleslas, 113, **113**
Biofeedback, 108-109, **108, 109**
Birth charts, 70-71, **70**
Blackmore, Dr. Susan, 17, 29, **29,** 33, 35
Blake, William, **39,** 56, **134**
Blavatsky, Mme. Helena, 88, **88**
Bloxham, Arnall, 52, 53, **53,** 54
Bond, Elijah J., 74
Book of the Dead, 42, 119
Bosch, Hieronymus, 130, **130, 131**

Bourges cathedral, France, **120**
Bouts, Dieric, **131**
Brain death, 21, **28,** 29
Brain scans, 29, **33**
Brazil, **65,** 82, 91
Britain, 91, **128,** 138
   NDE research, 20, 26
Broad, Prof. C. D., 81
Browning, Robert, **57**
Brown, John, 74, **75**
Brown, Rosemary, 82, 84, **84**
Bruno, Giordano, 56
Buddhism, 42-43, **42, 43,** 120, **132**
   Tibet, **38,** 44, **44,** 47, **47**
Burials, 41, 117-119, **119, 120-121,** 125
   live, 104, 105, 106, **106,** 110-111, 112
Burton, Julian, 92
Butts, Robert F., 86

C

Cabala, 45
Cambodia, 42
Campbell-Bannerman, Sir Henry, 141
Cancers, biofeedback, 109
Cannon, Alexander, 53, 55
Carrington, Hereward, **38**
Caste system, 60-61, **60, 61**
Cathari, 46
Catherine Labouré, St., 101
Catherine of Genoa, St., 101
Catherine of Siena, St., 101
Cayce, Edgar, 54, 70-71, 87, **87,** 88
Cemeteries, 118, 119, **119,** 125
Channelers, 86, 87, 88-89
Channeling (J. Klimo), 89
Channeling: How to Reach Out to Your Spirit Guides (K. Ridall), 89
Charbel Makhlouf, St., 101-102, **102**
Chelmsford witches, 53, **54**
China, 64, 74, **134,** 138
   burials, 119, **119,** 127, **127**
Chopin, Frédéric, **84**
Christianity, 29, **64, 70,** 71, 122
   afterlife, 119, 120, 124, **132, 133**
   cremation, 118
   early, 45, 46
Churchill, Winston, **94**
Church of Holy Innocents, Paris, 102
Church of St. John & Paul, Venice, 101
Church of the New Jerusalem, 125
Cinerary urn, **118**
Clive-Ross, Francis, 81-82
Coker, Nathan, 107
Colavida, Fernando, 50
Colburn, Nettie, 75, **75**
Coleridge, Samuel Taylor, 56
Collective unconscious, 128
Collyer, Anne, 96
Comas, 111
Concerning the Earths in Our Solar System (E. Swedenborg), 86
Congenital Erythropoietic Porphyria, 114
Conwell, Rev. Russell H., 92
Cook, Florence, **76**
Coombe-Tennant, Mrs. Winifred, 78, **80,** 81
Cove of Cork, Ireland, **53**
Crees, Romy, 48
Cremation, **46,** 118, 126
Cremation Society of England, 118
Crookall, Robert, 124, 125, 126
Crookes, Sir William, 75, 76
Cross-correspondence, 79, 82. *See also* Myers, Frederick W. H.
Crossley, Alan, 78
Cruz, Joan, 100
Cryptomnesia, 52, 53, 54, 66, 68
Cummins, Geraldine, 75, 81

D

Dalai lama, 47, **47**
Dali, Salvador, **56**
Darwin, Charles, 122, **122**
Day of the Dead, Mexico, 118, **118**
Death, 18, 20-21, 122-123, 140, 141
   celebration, 118, **118, 119**
   coincidence, 96-97
   incorruptibility, 99-103
   Victorian, **20**
"Death and the Gravedigger" (C. Schwabe), **135**
Defibrillators, 26, **28**
Dégas, Edgar, 85
Déjà vu, 68
Delirium tremens, 92
Demons, 130, **130, 131, 132**
   possession, **63, 64,** 67, **67**
"Descent into Limbo" (G. Bellini), **124**
Dharmapalas, 43
Dickens, Charles, 68, **68**
DNA (deoxyribonucleic acid), 129, **129**
Dr. Jekyll & Mr. Hyde (R. L. Stevenson), **66**
Dormouse, hibernating, **107**
Dorr, B. George, 80
Dracula (B. Stoker), 112
Dryden, Daisy, 20
Du Bourg, Anne, 141
Ducasse, C. J., 77
Duncan, Helen, 78, **78**
Dybbuks, 45

E

Eastland family, 49
Ebon, Martin, 68
Ecclesiastes 12 (Bible), **35**
Ectoplasm, **76, 77,** 78
Edison, Thomas A., 83, 141
Egypt, 42, 55, **67,** 106
   afterlife, 118, 119, 120, **120-121**
   mummification, 102, **102,** 118
   tomb paintings, **39, 120**
Electroencephalograms (EEG), 21, **28,** 35, 93
Electronic Voice Phenomenon (EVP), 83
Emerson, Ralph Waldo, 56
Encounters with the Past (J. Keeton), 53
England, 20, 29, 91, 118
Etruscans, **118, 125**
Europe, 42, 74, 111, 112
Evans, Jane, 52
Evolution in Two Worlds (C. Xavier), 82
Exorcism, **64,** 67, **67**
Extrasensory perception (ESP), 53, 54
   research, 77, 91-92, 97

F

Fakirs, 38, 104, **104**
Finney, Mrs. & Benja, 138
First World War, 97, **97**
Fleming, Mrs. Alice, 78
Flight 401, 94, **94**
Flint, Leslie, 126-127
Florence, Italy, **100**
Flournoy, Prof. Theodore, 86
Fontanelle, Bernard le Bovier de, 111
Ford, Henry, **56**
Fox, Catherine & Margaretta, 73-74, **74**
France, **64,** 91, 138

Franklin, Benjamin, 57
Frauds, 77, **77,** 78
Fraudulent Mediums Act, 1951, 78
Frohman, Charles, 140
From India to the Planet Mars (Prof. T. Flournoy), 86

G

Galatéri, Count Charles, 136
"Garden of Earthly Delights, The" (H. Bosch), 130, **130**
Garrett, Eileen, **65**
Gasparetto, Luiz Antonio, 82, 84, **85**
Gauguin, Eugène Henri Paul, **85**
Germany, 91, 112, 138
Ghosts. *See* Apparitions.
Giraldelli, Madame, **107**
Goethe, Johann Wolfgang von, 56
Granada, Spain, 47
Grant, Joan, 66
Greece, 65, 95, 111
   afterlife, 121, 123
   reincarnation, 43, 45
Green, Elmer & Alyce, 108, 109
Grey, Dr. Margot, 13, 14, 20, 26, **26,** 27-28
Gurney, Edmund, 97
Gyatso, Tentsin, 47

H

Haggard, Rider, 56
Haiti, 115, **115**
Hallowes, Odette, 32
Hallucinations, 33, 91-92, 93, 97
Hallucinogens, 39
Hamlet (W. Shakespeare), **92**
Hancock, John, 140, **140**
Haridas, 104
Harris, Barbara, 9-10, 13-14, 17
Harris, Melvin, 52
Harris, Rev. Doctor, 90
Hart, Dr. Hornell, 97
Hartley, Prof. Brian, 52
Harun-al-Rashid, **71**
Hawthorne, Nathaniel, 90, **90**
Hayes, Rutherford B., 141, **141**
Healing, 55, **55,** 108-109, **108**
Heaven, **20, 21,** 29, **36,** 130, **131-135,** 141
Heaven and Hell (E. Swedenborg), 86
Hebrews (Bible), 45
Hell, 27, 130, **130, 131-135**
Henrique, Mauricio, 83
Heredity, morphogenetic fields, 129
Hibernation, 107, **107**
Hill, Pamela, 111
Hinduism, **45,** 64, 121, **126, 133**
   castes, 60-61, **60, 61**
   cremation, 46, 126, **126**
   reincarnation, 42-43, **42,** 120
Hodgson, Dr. Richard, 80, 136
Holbein, Hans, **131**
Holland, Mrs., 80
Hollis-Billing, Mary, **89**
Holt, Dr. R. B., 124
Home, Daniel Dunglas, 74-75, **75**
Homer, 123
Hong Kong, funeral, **119**
Horoscopes, **61,** 70-71, **70-71**
Horst, Georg Conrad, 112
Houdini, Harry (E. Weiss), 105, **105**
Hugo, Victor, **56,** 140, **140**
Human Personality & its Survival of Bodily Death (F. W. H. Myers), 136
Humbolt, Friedrich, 140

Hunter, William, 140
Huxtable, Graham, 53
Hypnagogic images, 33
Hypnosis, 50-51, **51**, 55, **55**

I

Ibibio territory, Cameroon, 106
Incorruptibility, 99-103, **100**, **101**,
    102, **103**
Incorruptibles, The (J. Cruz), 100
India, 29, 60-61, **60**, **61**, 64
    holy men, 38, 104, **104**, 106
    reincarnation, 42-43, **42**, **43**
International Association for
    Near-death Experiences, 139
Inuits, afterlife, 121, **121**
Ireland, 53
Islam, symbolism, **42**, 46
Isle of Wight, 74, 95, **95**
Issels, Dr. Josef, 32

J

"Jacob's Dream" (W. Blake), **134**
James IV, King, 66, **66**
James, William, 80, 109, **109**
Japan, **43**, 64, **67**, 109, **113**
Jatakas (tales), 43
Jayavarman VII, **42**
Jenkins, Sarah Jean, 58
Jerome, St., 45
Jesus, **64**
Johnson, Alice, 78
Johnson, Martha, 35
John the Baptist, St., **101**
Judaism, 45, 64, **135**
Judas, **134**
Judgment after death, 119-121, **120**,
    124, **126**, 127, **134**
Jung, Carl Gustav, 56, **128**
Jürgenson, Friedrich, 83

K

Kahlbutz, Christian, 101, **101**
Kamiya, Joe, 109
Kampehl, Berlin, 101
Kanner, Dr. A., 110
Kant, Immanuel, 56
Keene, M. Lamar, **77**
Keeton, Joe, 53
Kelsey, Dr. Denys, 55
Khan, Durdana, **20**, 36, **36**
King, George, 88
King, William Lyon Mackenzie, 75
Kinski, Klaus, **114**
"Kiss of Vampire" (B. Biegas), **113**
Klimo, Jon, 89
Knickerbocker, Cholly, 141
Knight, J. Z., 86, 88, 89, **89**
Kreutziger, Sarah A., 10, 13, 22

L

Ladroni, Maria Anna, 100
Lamas, Tibet, **38**, 44, 47, **47**
"Last Judgement, The"
    (H. Bosch), **131**
    (S. Lochner), **133**
    (L. van Leyden), **126**
    (R. van der Weyden), **134**

Lawrence, Thomas Edward, 141, **141**
Lennon, John, **89**
Licorice, **121**
Life after Life (Dr. R. Moody), 20, **22**
Life at Death (Dr. K. Ring), 23, 32
Lill, John, 82
Lincoln, President & Mrs. A., 75, **75**
Link, The (M. Manning), 84
Little Ursulines Convent, **64**
Living apparitions, 95
Lloyd George, David, **56**
Lochner, Stefan, **133**
"Locked-in" syndrome, 111
Lodge, Sir Oliver, 76, **76**, 125-126
Loft, Bob (pilot), **94**
London, England, 28, 97, **138**
Longfellow, Henry Wadsworth, **126**
Lorenz, Paulo & Emilia, **70**
Los Angeles, California, survey, 92
Loudun, France, 64
Lourdes, France, 100
Lucas van Leyden, **126**
Lugosi, Bela, **112**
Lyttelton, Mary Catherine, 82

M

Macaire, Robert, **51**
MacLaine, Shirley, **88**
Magnetic resonance image (MRI), **29**
Mahler, Gustav, 56
Mandrake roots, **39**
Manichaeism, 45
Manning, Matthew, 84, **84**
Mann, Tad, 71
Marché des Innocents, Paris, 102
Marconi, Guglielmo, 83, **83**
Mary, Queen of Scots, **140**
Massacre of Jews, York, UK, 52, **52**
Mattei, Nadia, 103
Mazarin, Cardinal, **64**
McGregor, Geddes, 46
Medicine men, 38, 121, **121**
Mediums, 65, **65**, 74-81, 88, **88**.
    See also Channelers; Psychics.
Melville, Herman, 56
Mesopotamia, 119, 120
Mexico, 114, 118, **118**
Michel, Anneliese, 67
Middle East, 45, 60
Miller, Neal, 109
Mind Out of Time (I. Wilson), 55
Mit Damsis, Egypt, **67**
Mithraism, 45
Modigliani, Amedeo, **85**
Monroe, Robert, 34
Montségur, France, 46
Moody, Dr. Raymond, 13, 17, 20, **22**,
    26
Mortification of the flesh, 104,
    106-107
Moses, Rev. Stainton, 88, **88**
Mozart, Wolfgang Amadeus, **129**
Muldoon, Sylvan, **38**
Müller, Catherine Elise, 86, **86**
Mumler, William, 75
Mummification, 102-103, **102**, **103**,
    118, **120**
Murphy, Bridey, 50, 53
Music, psychic, 82, **84**
Myers, Frederic W. H., 78, 80, **80**, 97,
    136, 137
Mythopoeic faculty, 53, 54

N

Narcisse, **115**
Native Americans, 38, 88, 121, **121**

Neanderthals, 117
Near-death experiences (NDE), 10,
    13-14, 17, 18, 20
    core experience, 20-21, 24-25
    life transformation, 21, 25, 28, 31
    negative, 26, 27, 28
Nevers, France, **100**
New Age Movement. *See* Channelers.
New Science of Life, A (R.
    Sheldrake), 129
New York, 73, 112
Nichiren Buddhism, **67**
Nigeria, shamans, 65, **65**
Nirvana, 43, **43**, 44, 120
Nosferatu, the Vampyre (movie), **114**
Nunes, José, 83

O

Odor of sanctity, 100
Ono, Yoko, **89**
Origen, 45
Orphics, 43
Osel, Lama, 47, **47**
Osis, Kalis, 92
Oslo, Norway, 94
Ouija boards, 74, **74**, 86
Out-of-body experience (OBE), 24-25,
    32-35, 38, **38-39**
Ovid, 68

P

Palmer, John, 141
Palmerston, Lord, 141, **141**
Palm Sunday Case, The, 81
Papua New Guinea, 102
Paradise, **20**, 21, 29, **36**, 130, **131-135**,
    141
Paramnesia, 68
Park, John, 124-125
Patton, Jr. Gen G. S., **57**
Peacocks, **42**
Pelletier, Blessed Marie de
    Sainte-Euphrasie, 103
Persia (now Iran), **46**, 119
Personalities, multiple, 53, 61, 66, **66**
Phantasms of the Living (SPR), 96
Phobias, 55
Phone Calls from the Dead (D. Scott
    Rogo & R. Bayless), 83
Photographs, spirit, **75**, 76, **88**
"Physical Detection of the Astral
    Body" *Theta* magazine (C. S.
    Alvarado), 124
Picasso, Pablo, 84, **84**
Picknett, Lynn, 34
Piddington, J. G., 80
Pindar, 45
Piper, Mrs. Leonora, 78, **80**
Planchette boards, 74
Plato, 45, 123, **123**
Plutarch, 118
Podmore, Frank, 80
Pollock, John & Florence, 59
Polynesia, 121
Possession, 62, 63, **63**, 64-67, **64**, **65**
Post-Mortem Journal (J. Sherwood),
    141
Powell, Robert, 71
Price, Lily, 124
Principles of Psychology, The (W.
    James), 109
Projection of the Astral Body, The (S.
    Muldoon & H. Carrington), 38
Psychics, 76, 82-84, **82**, **83**, **84**, **85**
Pursel, Jach, 89
Pythagorus, 45

R

Radagast, Pat, 89
Rais, Gilles de (Black Baron), 114
Ramdasji, Shri, 106
Rameses I, **102**
Rasputin, Grigori, 106, **106**
Raudive, Dr. Konstantin, 83, **83**
Rawlings, Dr. Michael, 26, 27-28
Reflections on Life after Life (Dr.
    R. Moody), 20
Regression therapy, 52, 53-55, **55**
Reincarnation, 41-47, 56, **56**, **57**,
    58-61, 120
    spiritualism, 128
    symbolism, 42, **42**, **43**, 44.
    See also Astrology; Hypnosis;
    Possession.
Reincarnation as a Christian Hope
    (G. McGregor), 46
*Reincarnation in the Twentieth
    Century* (M. Ebon), 68
Religions, 21, 23, 28, 29
    afterlife, 130, **132**, **133**, **134**,
    135
    astral flight, 38, **38-39**
    reincarnation, 42-47
Remote viewing, 34
Renoir, Pierre Auguste, **85**
Repo, Don (flight engineer), **94**
Republic (Plato), 123
Research, 60-61, 77, 108-109
    apparitions, 91-92, 97
    biofeedback, 108-109
    NDE, 20-21, 22-29
Réunion, **67**
Rhine, Dr. J. B., 77, 91
Rhine, Dr. Louisa, 97
Richmond, Mrs. Zoe, 125-126
Ridall, Kathryn, 89
Ring, Dr. Kenneth, 20, **22**, 23, 25, 26,
    32
Ritchie, George, 18, 20
Rituals, 118, 119, **128**
Roberts, Jane, 86, 89
Robertson, Marc, 70, **70-71**, 71
Rochas, Albert de, 50, 55
Roff, Mary, 62, 64, **64**
Rogo, D. Scott, 20, 22, 27, 31
    telephone calls from the dead,
    82-83, 83
Roman Empire, 45, 95, **110**
Rome, Italy, 103
Rossetti, Dante Gabriel, **57**
Rousseau, Jean-Jacques, 122
Royalty, spiritualism, 74
Russell, Bertrand, **71**

S

Sabom, Dr. Michael B., 10, 13, 14, 17,
    20, 22, 26
Sacks, Dr. Oliver, 111
Sailor's life, Napoleonic wars, 53, **54**
"St. Dominic Presides over the
    Burning of Heretics" (P.
    Berruguete), 46
St. Mary's, Castlegate, York, UK, 52
Sallust, 45
Sanchi, India, 43
Sanni yakuma, 67
Saponification, 102-103
Saturn, **70-71**, 71
Sàvoca, Sicily, **103**
Schatzman, Dr. Morton, 93, **93**
Schiele, Egon, **27**
Schimmelpenninck, Mary-Anne, 141
Schreiber, Klaus, **83**
Schulz, Dr. Johannes, 109
Schwabe, Carlos, **135**

Séances, 65, 74-77, 138, **138**
Seth, **86**, 89
Shaka Muni, **43**
Shamans, 38, **38**, 65, **65**, 86
Shankar, Ravi, 60-61
Sheldrake, Rupert, 129, **129**
Shelley, Percy Bysshe, 56
Sherwood, Jane, 141
Shock treatment, 21, **21**, 26, **28**
Sibelius, Jean, 56
Siberia, **38**, **86**
Sidgwick, Henry, 91, **91**
Signorelli, Luca, **132**
Silver cord, **34-35**, 124, 125
Simeon Stylites, St., **106**, 107, **107**
Sitwell, Dame Edith, **56**
Skeletons, Day of the Dead, **118**
Skeptical Inquirer, 89
Sleeping Prophet, The (J. Stearn), 87
Sleeping sickness, 111, **111**
Smith, Hélène, 86, **86**
Society for Psychical Research (SPR), 28, 80, 91, 96, 138
"Soul Hovering Above the Body, The" (W. Blake), **39**
Southeast Asia, 60
Speaking Across the Borderline (F. Heslop), 124-125
Spinelli, Dr. Ernesto, 94
Spirits materialization, **76**, **77**, 78
Spiritualism, 73-83, 88, 91
    afterlife, 117, 122, 124-125, 126-128.
    See also Art, psychic; Channelers.
Sri Lanka, **45**, 60, 65, 67, **67**, **106**
Stark, Dr. Mortis, 50
Stearn, Jess, 87
Steiner, Rudolf, 70
Stevens, Dr. E. Winchester, 62
Stevenson, Prof. Ian, 49, 60, **60**, 66, 70, 97, 138
Stevenson, Robert Louis, **66**
Stewart, Mrs. A. J., 66, **66**
Stoker, Bram, 112
Stone Age, graves, 41, 117
Stromberg, Gustav, 56
    Stylites, 107

Supreme Adventure, The (R. Crookall), 125, 126
Surveys, 91-92, 96, 139
Survival pacts, 136, 137-139
Swann, Ingo, **34**
Swan on a Black Sea (G. Cummins), 81
Swedenborg, Emanuel, 86, 125, **125**
Syria, 106-107

T

Table rapping, 138, **138**
Takster, China, 47
Tart, Dr. Charles, 35
Techniques of Astral Projection, The (R. Crookall), 124
Tellneshin (Antakya, Turkey), 107
Temple decoration, **44**, **45**
Temporal lobe epilepsy, 68, 92
Tenuto, William, **89**
Teresa Margaret of the Sacred Heart, St., 100-101, **100**
Teresa of Avila, St., **100**, 101
Terry, Ellen, 127
Theatre Royal, London, **94**
Thomas, Theodore, 140
Thomason, Sarah Grey, 89
Thompson, Alex, 37
Thornton, Penny, 70, 71
Thouless, Dr. Robert, 138, **138**, 139
Thurston, Father Herbert, 101
Tibet, 38, **38**, **43**, 44, **44**, 47, **47**
Tighe, Virginia Burns, 50, 53, **53**
Tlingits, Alaska, 61
Togo, West Africa, **115**
Tomb guardian, T'ang dynasty, **127**
Tombs, Egypt, **39**, 42, **120**
Torres, Osel Hita, 47, **47**
Torres, Penny, 88
Toulouse-Lautrec, Henri, **85**
Trances, 65, **65**, 75, 84, **85**, 87

Treasurer's House, York, UK, 95, **95**
Tree of life, **46**, 118
Turcott, Marjorie, 89

U

Unfinished Symphonies (R. Brown), **84**
Upanishads, 42
Ur, Royal Cemetery, 119, **119**
USA, 20, 26, 74, 75, 83, 91

V

Vampire Cat of Nabeshima, **113**
Vampires, 112-114
Varanasi, India, **46**, **61**
Venice, Italy, 101
Vennum, Lurancy, 62, 64, **64**
Verrall, Margaret & Helen, 78, 80
Vianney, St. Jean Baptiste Marie, **101**
Victoria, Queen, 74, **75**
Vieira, Dr. Waldo, 82
Vienna, Austria, 111
Vikings, Isle of Wight, **95**
Virgil, 45, 123
Virgini, Lieut. M., 136
Vishnu, **45**
Vision of Tundale, 119
Voltaire, 56
Voodoo worship, 65, 115, **115**

W

Wade, Sir Claude, 104
Wagner, Richard, 56
Waldorf, Ginger, 58
Waterhouse, Joan, 53, **54**, 55
Watseka Wonder case, 62, 64

Weiss, Erich (H. Houdini), 105, **105**
Weyden, Rogier van der, **134**
Wheel of Life, 44, **44**
White, Dr. & Mrs., 95
Whitman, Walt, 56, **57**
Wiertz, Antoine, **55**
Williams, Louise, 48
Wilson, Ian, 10, 20, 55, **60**, 61, 66
Witchcraft, **39**, 53, **54**, 55, 78
Witchcraft Act, 1735, 78
Withers, Frank (Seth), 86, **86**
Wofford, Dorothy, 66
Woolger, Roger, 55
Woolley, Sir Leonard, 119
Wordsworth, William, 56
Writing, automatic, 75, 79, **79**, 82-83, **83**, 125
    channelers, 86, 87, 88-89
    F. W. H. Myers, 78, 80-81, 137

X

Xavier, Candido (Chico), 82, **82**, 83
Xenophanes, 45

Y

Yeshe, Lama, 47
Yogis, 104, **104**, 106, **106**, 107
York, England, 52, **52**, 95, **95**

Z

Zen Buddhism, **43**
Zola, Émile, **110**
Zombies, 115, **115**
Zoroaster, 45, 119-120
Zwingli, Huldrych, 140

PHOTOGRAPHIC SOURCES

AA Picture Library: 95tl; **Bryan and Cherry Alexander**: 121br; **Ancient Art and Architecture Collection**: 39tr, cr, br; **Archiv für Kunst und Geschichte**: 101b, 131br; **Associated Press**: 53c; **John Beckett**: 77bc, cr; **Musées Royaux des Beaux-Arts de Belgique** (photo: G. Cussac): 55b; **Dr. Susan Blackmore**: 22t, b, 29b; **Bodleian Library**: 39c; **Bridgeman Art Library**: 27, 46tr, 57tl, 60bl, 61bl, br, 75tl, 79 inset, 84bl (Giraudon), 85tr (Lauros Giraudon), 94tr, 97 (Imperial War Museum), 124t, 126b, 130r, 131tl, bl (Giraudon), 132tr, 133t, 134tc, r, 135tl; **British Library**: 21l, 134bc; **British Museum**: 119bl; **Robert F. Butts**: 86tl; **Romano Cagnoni**: 115t; **Edgar Cayce Foundation Archives**: 87r; **Jean-Loup Charmet**: 39b, 51r, 111r, 113cr, 114tr; **Bruce Coleman Ltd**: 39cl (N.G. Blake), 88b (K. Balcomb); **C.M. Dixon**: 43l, 45t, bl, 127b, 134bl; **Mary Evans Picture Library**: 38tl, bl, br, 39tc, 52, 56br, 63r, 64br, 65tr (Soc. for Psychical Research), 66l, 67tr, 68l, 71b, 74t, c, 75b, 76tr (Soc. for Psychical Research), br (Psychic Press), 78 (Harry Price Collection, University of London), 79r (College for Psychic Studies), 80t, c (Soc. for Psychical Research), 81t, 82t, br & 83tl (G.L. Playfair), tr (M. Cassirer), 84bc & br (G.L. Playfair), 86bl, 88tr, 89tl, 90l, 95b, 100tl, tr, 104tr, 105r (Harry Price Collection), 106t, bl (Harry Price Collection), 107tr, 109b (Soc. for Psychical Research), 110t, 122b, 124b, 129b (Explorer), 135tr, 138t, b, 140bl, 141bl; **Werner Forman Archive**: 101tr, cr, 103tl, 106br, 107tl, 110b; **Fortean Picture Library**: 100cl, cr, b, 101tl, 102l; **Michael Freeman**: 42l, 46bl; **Glasgow Museums & Art Galleries**: 140t; **Sally and Richard Greenhill**: 119br; **Margot Grey**: 26t; **Sonia Halliday**: 64bl, 123; **Robert Harding Picture Library**: 55t (T. Mercer), 65br, 103tr, b; **Rainer Holbe**: 83br; **Michael Holford**: 42r, 43br, 45br, 46br, 118tl, 119t, bc, 120, 121t, 125, 133br; **Hulton-Deutsch Collection**: 57br, 71t, c, 83c, 94br, 104tl; **Hutchison Library**: 38tr (C. Preire), 43tr, 44r, 46cl, 60tl (A. Hill), 65l (Camera Pix), bl & 126tl (M. McIntyre); **Image Bank**: 87tl, br, 93r, 108b (M. St. Gil); **Images Colour Library**: 61t, 76bl, 92t, 132c, br; **Imperial War Museum**: 141r; **Dr. A.G. Khan**: 20tr, c, b; **J.Z. Knight**: 89tr; **Kobal Collection**: 112l, br, 114tl; **Kunsthistorisches Museum, Vienna**: 112tr; **His Grace the Archbishop of Canterbury and the Trustees of Lambeth Palace Library**: 54t; **Raymond Mander and Joe Mitchenson Theatre Collection**: 20tl; **Mansell Collection**: 53t; **Mexicolore**: 118bl, br; **Mountain Camera**: 39tl (John Cleare), 44l (Colin Monteath); **National Portrait Gallery, London**: 56t, 57cr, bl, 141tl; **The Nelson Museum, Monmouth**: 54b; **Peter Newark's Pictures**: 126tr, 140br; **Octopus Publishing Group Ltd./Constantino Reyes-Valerio**: 118tr; **Oxford Scientific Films**: 107br (O. Newman), 114bl (S. Dalton); **Ann and Bury Peerless**: 133bl; **Photographers International**: 66c; **Picturepoint**: 53b; **Popperfoto**: 56bl, 57tr, 104b, 106c; **Psychic Press**: 75tr; **Dr. Mauro Pucciarelli**: 135bl; **Rex Features**: 88tl (LGI Photo Agency/D. Dubler), 89b (K. Shinoyama), 122tl (SIPA); **Adrian Rowland**: 93l; **Science Photo Library**: 21r & 26c (A. Hart Davis), r (D. Leah), 28l (A. Tsiaras), 29t (CNRI), 33r (Dr. J. Mazziotta et al), 129 background & tr (P. Menzel); **Scottish National Portrait Gallery/Private Collection**: 66r; **Dr. Rupert Sheldrake**: 129l; **Brian Snellgrove**: 84tl, tr, c, 85tc, cr, bl, bc, br; **Cecil Beaton photograph, courtesy of Sotheby's London**: 56cr; **Frank Spooner Pictures/Gamma**: 46tl (X. Zimbardo), 47t (M. Gonzales), b (T. Stoddart), 56cl (Socias-Cover), 60tr (L. Skodgfors), 67tl (B. Iverson), bl (R. Gaillarde), 85tl (A. Morvan), 109t (K. Kurita), 115c (D. Laine), b (J.C. Francolon); **Roy Stemman**: 34t; **Ingo Swann**: 34b; **Syndication International**: 77b, 80b; **From 'The Forces of Destiny' by Penny Thornton**: 70tl, bl; **Topham Picture Source**: 128t; **UPI/Bettmann, New York**: 94l; **Staatmuseum für Volkerkunde**: 86r; **Photo Vatican Museums**: 116-7; **Ian Wilson**: 60br; **ZEFA**: 102tr (Thiele), b & 107bl (Havlicek), 127t.

b - bottom; c - center; t - top; r - right; l - left.

Efforts have been made to contact the holder of the copyright for each picture. In several cases these have been untraceable, for which we offer our apologies.

Reader's Digest Fund for the Blind is publisher of the Large-Type Edition of *Reader's Digest*. For subscription information about this magazine, please contact Reader's Digest Fund for the Blind, Inc., Dept. 250, Pleasantville, N.Y. 10570.